Excerpts from
HOW JUICES RESTORE HEAL

How fortunate you picked up this book, for ... renewed health and a lifetime of fulfilled vibrancy. Gone will be those sick headaches, that dragging fatigue, that gnawing depression.

(chapter 1)

* * *

Our food is a hazard to our health! Examine your own daily eating habits. How much of your food that you eat daily has been refined, processed, degraded, manipulated, machined, mauled or mangled and then cooked to death? (chapter 3)

* * *

A man is as old as his blood vessels. Many people with arthritis suffer from fragile capillaries. (chapter 5)

* * *

I tried various juice drink combinations and only after several months did I discover what worked best for me. Here is my personal formula for that GOLDEN GLOW. (chapter 7)

* * *

Arthritis is not inherited. What you may inherit are the poor eating habits of your parents. (chapter 9)

* * *

Raw vegetable juices are a goldmine to anyone who is suffering from ulcers and colitis. (chapter 10)

* * *

Here are some basic guidelines to follow to successfully fight the battle of the bulge for the rest of your life. (chapter 11)

* * *

It is **NOT** a fact that one's normal blood pressure should be 100 plus the individual's age. (chapter 12)

* * *

The prostate is often the seat of disorders which often end in surgical correction. Sometimes the "cure" is worse than the problem.(chapter 13)

* * *

More nerve cells are devoted to serving our sense of sight than are devoted to any of our other senses. Therefore, it is important that these nerve cells are constantly bathed in proper nourishment. (chapter 14)

All this and much more you will find in the 17 chapters of HOW JUICES RESTORE HEALTH NATURALLY.

HOW JUICES
RESTORE HEALTH
NATURALLY

by
SALEM KIRBAN

First Printing..April, 1980
Second Printing...March, 1981

Published by SALEM KIRBAN, Inc., Kent Road, Huntingdon
Valley, Pennsylvania, 19006. Copyright © 1980 by Salem Kirban.
Printed in the United States of America. All rights reserved, in-
cluding the right to reproduce this book or portions thereof in any
form.
ISBN 0-912582-30-8
Library of Congress Catalog Card No. 78-70259

ACKNOWLEDGMENTS

To **Doreen Frick,** who carefully proofread the text.

To **Koechel Designs,** for creating the artwork for the front and back covers.

To **John E. Peterson,** of Koechel Designs, for taking the color photographs of the juice combinations.

To **Walter W. Slotilock,** Chapel Hill Litho, for skillfully making all the illustration negatives.

To **Batsch Company,** for excellent craftsmanship in setting the type.

To **Bethany Press,** for printing with all possible speed and quality.

Note

DEDICATION

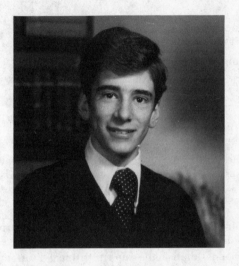

To our son

DUANE M. KIRBAN

who discovered
that live juices
do play an important role
in restoring
and maintaining full, vibrant health.

WHY I WROTE THIS BOOK

It was October 13, 1976. I was addressing a congregation of some 700 people at the Wednesday night service of the Anchorage Baptist Temple in Anchorage, Alaska.

Before introducing me, Pastor Jerry Provo asked this vast audience:

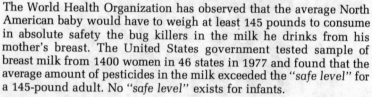

> How many people in this audience can really say they are healthy . . . raise your hands.

After a brief moment, he observed:

> I see only 20-25 hands raised. This proves that this message by Salem Kirban is needed.

The World Health Organization has observed that the average North American baby would have to weigh at least 145 pounds to consume in absolute safety the bug killers in the milk he drinks from his mother's breast. The United States government tested sample of breast milk from 1400 women in 46 states in 1977 and found that the average amount of pesticides in the milk exceeded the "safe level" for a 145-pound adult. No "safe level" exists for infants.

By weaning our children on the same nutritional disasters we take into our bodies, we guarantee that we will bequeath these same sins to the next generation. We are living in a (legal and illegal) drug-oriented society. We have sacrificed common sense on the altar of expediency and profit.

Dr. Robert Bruce, a medical doctor, geneticist and physicist who works in Toronto with the Ontario Cancer Institute, says that food is the No. 1 cause of human cancer in North America. Dr. A. B. Miller, director of epidemiology with the Canadian Cancer Society of Toronto says that 50% of "common cancers"—cancers of the intestine, breast and bladder —are directly related to the food people eat.

A lady in Southampton, Pennsylvania remarked to me:

> It's awful to watch someone you love die knowing they won't try the nutritional way.

That's why I wrote this book! To help save lives!

Salem Kirban

Huntingdon Valley, Pennsylvania
U.S.A. January 1980

CONTENTS

1

HOW JUICES GAVE ME
TEENAGE VIBRANCY AT AGE 50

**Beauty
Begins
Within**

Now! You can enter the wonderful world of juices . . . and feel young again!

How fortunate that you picked up this book, for it can start you on the road to renewed health and a lifetime of fulfilled vibrancy.

Gone will be those sick headaches, that dragging fatigue, that gnawing depression. This book will be your guide to the healing and regenerative powers of natural energy — raw juices!

You will not find beauty and health in lotions and creams that only cover up the ravages of Mother Nature and reveal the lines of time.

Your new life can begin now . . . this very week if you discover the secret that took me 50 years to accept!

The daily use of fresh live juices can change your life. It can make you a new person physically. It may be the answer to the headaches, the arthritic pains, circulation problems or any other of the myriad ailments that may plague you.

**At 50
I Faced
Reality**

At 50 years of age I was going downhill fast, physically. I was aware of it . . . yet I did not know how to cope with this problem.

I went to my physician annually and took a complete physical. I was told that for a man of 50 I was in good shape. "For a man of 50," that's when I began to wonder. <u>If I felt this bad at 50 . . . how would I feel at 55?</u>

**My Body
Was Trying
To Tell
Me Something**

My hair was turning grey. I would go to bed tired and wake up tired. I was a compulsive eater, snacking at the wrong times. Day to day problems worried me. I had a host of mysterious ailments. Whether these ailments were imaginary or real . . . only time would tell. But I knew enough about the human body to know that these signs were potential warning signals.

And I was ignoring the blinking red lights!

How odd! Here I was a student of the Bible, aware of the dietary laws of the Old Testament yet not coming face to face with reality as to what the human body requires.

**How I
Became a
New Man**

It was quite by accident that a minister friend of mine introduced me to Dr. Carey Reams. Dr. Reams, a naturopath, made the "*lemon and distilled water fast*" popular. I went to his retreat in March, 1976 and came out a new man!

While the Reams system has been blasted by some in the medical profession and his retreat closed down . . . I will ever be grateful to him for introducing me to sound nutrition practices.

From this initial stepping stone of a new life from a 3-day fast at the Reams retreat. I was then schooled on the importance of **LIVE JUICES.**

I learned that **life sustains life.** Now I could understand how a diet of hamburgers, french fries, cola drinks and the standard American diet . . . were devoid of life. These dead foods could not possibly sustain life at its utmost.

Is it any wonder that even children become early victims of illness, exhibit despondency, inability to concentrate, and fatigue?

I am writing this book in July, 1978. Soon I will be 53 years of age. My nutrition program began at 50. In the last 3 years I have made intensive studies of nutrition. (I regularly receive all the major medical publications, the natural health publications and special drug newsletters.)

The Most Important Paragraph In This BOOK!

If someone were to ask me what is the one most important fact I have learned in these three years THAT TURNED MY LIFE AROUND, I would unhesitatingly say:

THE IMPORTANCE OF DRINKING LIVE JUICES <u>DAILY</u>

I cannot overemphasize this point. I practice this in my own life. I can attest to its effectiveness. IT WORKS FOR ME. It can work for you.

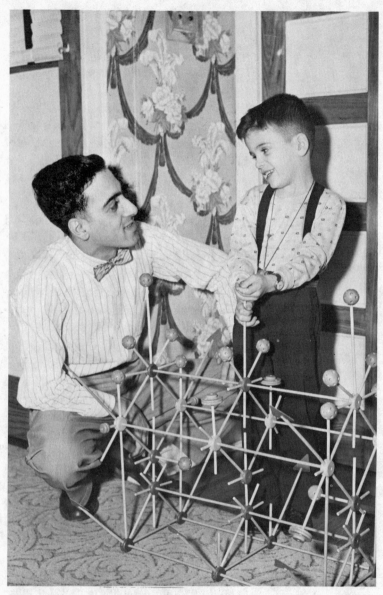

This photo, taken in 1952, shows author with son, Dennis, engaged in building a house with Tinker toys. As a house needs a firm foundation so does the human body. Live juices provide that firm foundation that can help insure continued good health.

The daily drinking of live juices has honestly changed my life! My fatigue has vanished. Rarely do I get a headaches ... perhaps once or twice a year (and that is only when, while travelling, I am off my diet). Symptoms of illnesses that I once had ... have vanished. My creative ability has increased. My ability to meet problems head-on has increased. At 50 years of age I became a new person.

And I have continued to maintain this vibrant life because of daily use of FRESH LIVE JUICES.

It's Great To Wake Up With Energy!

I wake up fresh and alive in the morning ... abounding in energy. And the daily drinking of juices helps me maintain energy throughout the day.

My hair has become thicker and more lustrous. My skin has become more supple. My life has taken on new meaning and purpose.

I was so overjoyed at making this discovery that I wanted to share this good news with my friends and relatives. (And that can be a mistake.)

I have found one of the most difficult things to do is to convince those you love to follow the same live juice program that gave me back my youth.

I see them constantly plagued with colds and other problems ... trying to resolve them with all sorts of medication and antibiotics. And they have a tiger by the tail! Believe me ... it is hard to convince others

Life
Sustains
Life

of the fact that **LIFE SUSTAINS LIFE** . . . that fresh raw fruit and vegetable juices are nature's own lifeline!

Americans take over 100-million aspirin tablets a day. It is a billion-dollar business. And this is only the tip of the iceberg. More billions are spent on a host of standard prescriptions and patent medications.

How I wish that everyone reading this book would discover **THE IMPORTANCE OF DRINKING LIVE JUICES DAILY.** It could change your life this very week. It changed mine!

2

HOW JUICES CAN TURN YOUR STRESSES INTO STRENGTHS

The Lesson I Learned At a Campfire

One evening at a campfire meeting in the heart of a Virginia woods an important truth was conveyed very graphically to me.

As the fire blazed on the dark night, and you could hear the crackling of the logs I was captivated by the warm glow of the light.

Surrounding us were tall pine trees. And as I looked up I could see the sparks lifting off the campfire and soaring up to the heavens vanishing above the tall pines.

It was then that verse in Job 5:7 hit me:

> . . . man is born unto trouble,
> as the sparks fly upward.

This verse reminded me that just as sure as sparks fly upward from a fire . . . that is the certainty that each individual will face trouble throughout life.

I have found this to be true.

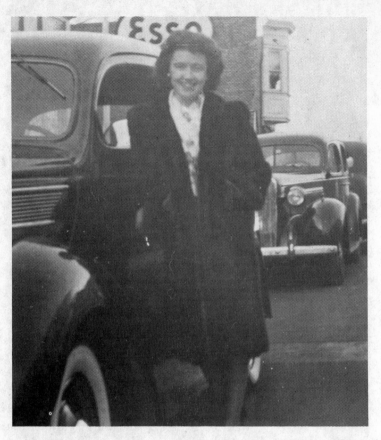

My sweetheart, Mary, gave me this photo in December, 1945, while I was in the Navy. She is standing beside her father's 1937 Ford on 8th Street in Philadelphia. Eight months later, Mary and I were married.

I look back on those days with warm memories. Life was less complicated. While life had its share of stresses, they were not as accelerated as they are today. The advent of television, jet planes and the drug culture has been responsible, in part, for contributing to the growing ills of a highly stressed populace.

Most people have lost the art of knowing how to relax, how to enjoy nature. It would appear that perhaps our greatest joys have become (1) making money, (2) spending money on luxuries and (3) paving everything that is green and placing a shopping center on top of it!

Perhaps it is time we realign our priorities in life . . . and like the old, slow 1937 Ford, adapt some old-fashioned ideas . . . some of which would include getting back to nature, start drinking live juices daily and stop eating junk foods.

I grew up during the Depression days of the 1930's and I matured quickly during my teenage years because I was in the U.S. Navy during World War 2.

I faced the normal stresses that young people faced in that day . . . plus a few more. My father died when I was one year old, and I was placed in an orphanage at 7. It was called Girard College. I can remember that first day my mother left me at Girard. I could not understand how she could leave me and travel 100 miles back to our hometown of Scranton, Pennsylvania. I cried for 3 solid days.

My Stresses Began Early in Life

Upon graduation from Girard I only had a few months of freedom when I was drafted and sent overseas.

While the stresses I faced in those early days of my youth were heartbreaking . . . I honestly believe the stresses that young and old alike face today are even more intense.

We are living in a stress environment. Our way of life has accelerated at a much faster pace since the early 1970's.

Young people are finding it difficult to cope with problems in and out of school. Adults are finding it difficult to provide for their family. And older people are finding their retirement years not a dream but a nightmare!

Everyone believes their problems are the biggest. It is my privilege to speak in hundreds of churches nationwide. And many people discuss their problems with me.

And to me, some of these problems appear so small that I would like to trade my problems for theirs.

But to them, their problem is a mountain. To you, it may appear like a molehill.

We are living in a day of stress. And world conditions will not improve. They will bring greater and greater stress to each of us. Why? Because of more shortages of vital raw materials such as oil and water. The mood of nations is changing. We are living in a world of increasing discontent ... discontent that erupts into wars, shortages, strikes and violence.

A Vicious Circle

Americans, particularly, have become highly materialistic. Husbands and wives now work and some even hold down two jobs ... trapped in a fast pace of living that taxes one's physical endurance.

Let me give you insight into my own life. I believe the Bible when God tells us to

> ... *cast all your care* [worries] *upon Him; for He careth for you.*
> (1 Peter 5:7)

And it is easy for me to quote this to a friend when he has a real problem. Believe me it is far more difficult to follow. Why? Because we are human. We are not perfect. We strive to have a life worry-free, free from trials and tensions. But in this world we can never achieve that ultimate goal.

Right now I am under tremendous stress.

I am working on three books. I must finish writing this book this week.

Besides that I am creating and publishing a new Reference Edition of the Bible. This means I have to write commentary notes for over 1000 pages of this Bible. And I must design and put this entire 2000 page Bible together, proofread it and publish it. This is a mammoth undertaking for one individual to take on. (A new Bible is generally undertaken by a staff of 10 or more people who work on the project for years). Yet I must publish this Bible within 4 months. And to add to my stress, my bank turned down my request for a "work in process" loan to meet the heavy expenses in creating this work!

Learning To Live With Stress

That's part of my stress. This coming week, I have to fly to the West Coast, speak 5 times within 4 days . . . each time about 1 hour long plus put on a One-Day Seminar for ministers where I'll be speaking for 7 hours.

On top of that I direct a publishing company and a non-profit organization and must keep both afloat so we can pay our bills . . . in spite of the fact that postal rates are escalating and prices on everything are going sky high.

Yet I must take time to work in my garden, fellowship with my family, answer mail, and resolve daily problems of running a business.

Stress?

I have plenty of it . . . every day. And from a physical standpoint I would have had a nervous breakdown long ago if I had con-

**The Key
To Combating
Stress**

tinued my regular eating habits. I could honestly have never made it.

What turned my stress into strength? Two things: my faith and live juices!

LIVE JUICES can turn your stresses into strengths, too. But you will never know until you try them!

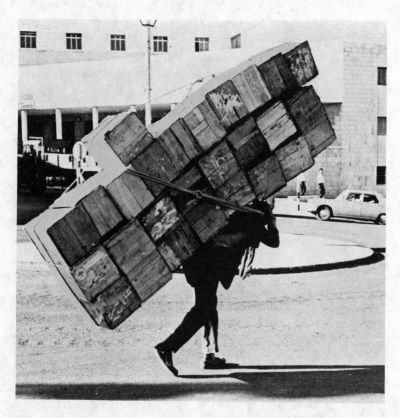

Stop carrying all your problems on your back. Live one day at a time. Remember, no matter how great your problem: "This, too, shall pass!" Stress rapidly depletes the nutrients in your body. Live juices can replace them quickly!

3

HOW 3 SQUARE MEALS A DAY
CAN SEND YOU TO AN EARLY GRAVE

**Growing Up
On Salads**

Our food is a hazard to our health!

From time immemorial, people have expressed love one for another through the sharing of food. My family comes from Lebanon. And in the Middle East it is the custom to serve every visitor a meal.

Those meals were nutrition-high meals. Generally my mother would make a salad brimming over with parsley, mint leaves and assorted greens and soaking in a garlic-smothered olive oil.

Today we have sacrificed common sense to sugar-coated sensation. We are eating too much of the foods that hurt us and far too little of the foods that help us.

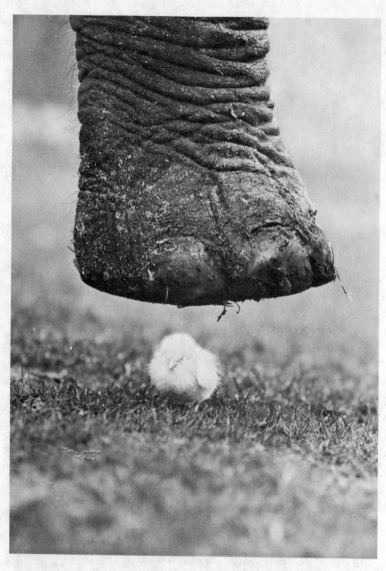

Many people pride themselves in the fact that they have been eating junk foods all their life and are still "healthy." But, like the chick pictured above, they are living under a time bomb of impending doom. You can't fool Mother Nature! After years of feeding your body junk, one day the specter of illness will lower its crushing foot!

**Our Children
Adopt Our
Bad Eating
Habits**

And the tragedy of it all is that we are weaning our children on the same nutritional disasters. This almost guarantees that they will suffer the same illnesses that will afflict us.

I can never understand how parents can claim they love their children . . . yet feed them junk foods that will either send them to a premature grave or sow the seed for a host of future ailments.

I'm a firm believer in following good, sound health practices. I believe that most of the people in hospitals are there because of neglect of their body . . . self-inflicted diseases. You can make yourself well or ill. It depends, for a major part, on the food you consume. And millions of individuals are, perhaps unconsciously, slowly committing suicide at their own tables!

**Our Bodies
Are a Gift
From God**

The word <u>health</u> comes from the old English word _hailo_ (or kailo) — meaning whole and complete. From this same root word we derive the modern word, <u>holy.</u>

What we are doing is separating the concept of God from health and further separating the concept of health from the food we eat. We are told simply to _"eat three square meals a day."_

In today's world . . . this is impossible. Most of our food is de-vitalized before it is consumed. One might as well eat sawdust. Our food is loaded with chemicals. And to this we cook it to death . . . thus changing the natural properties of the food.

It was Seneca who said:

Man does not die . . . he kills himself.

Some people attribute disease to the devil. In the New Testament we are told that our body is the Temple of the Holy Spirit. (1 Corinthians 6:19).

Yet we proceed to treat it like a garbage can . . . daily! Is it any wonder we are constantly sick; perhaps not sick enough to go to the hospital . . . but sick enough to be on one medication or another . . . popping pills, fighting fatigue and depression and tension headaches.

Life Begins With Live Juices

Now I don't want to minimize the importance of your physician. I believe he is a very important arm of the healing arts. And certainly no change in diet should be made without consulting with him.

I am sure he would be the first to agree that you give up junk foods and start eating live foods. And I would hope he would recommend that you drink _live_ juices daily.

By live juices I do not mean canned juice or orange juice or V-8 type juice. I mean taking fresh celery, carrots, string beans, etc. and juicing them through a juicer and drinking them immediately.

And (for an adult) I do not mean drinking a 4 or 6 ounce glass daily . . . but at least 24 ounces daily!

I am not going to make a rash statement and say that by drinking live juices every day you will resolve all your physical

**Nutrition
Before
Drugs**

problems. I can't say that. Much depends on what medication you are taking, how far along your present illness has progressed . . . and whether the nutrients from live juices can filter to your entire body.

(Chemotherapy and other drastic methods sometimes neutralize the ability of nutrients to reach vital, afflicted areas.)

But I do believe in the basic concept that life sustains life . . . that is live foods and live juices are what are urgently needed . . . daily, to sustain life and to help you live life on its highest plane. How long would an automobile survive on junk oil and dirt-encrusted spark plugs and a carburetor with narrowing orifices?

**Let's
Realign
Our
Priorities**

What I am saying is that we take better care of our house, our car, our golf clubs, our clothes . . . which are all replaceable . . . than we do with our body. Yet our body is the only one we get in this world!

Be honest with yourself! Isn't that true. Then you give yourself a false re-assurance saying to your family:

Well, we eat three square meals a day.

We feed animals better than we feed ourselves. We gorge ourselves on health-destroying hamburgers, smothered with junk and sandwiched with soggy rolls that are sure to clog our colon.

Women will buy all types of moisturizers

Change
Your
Eating Habits

when one or two tablespoons of safflower oil will moisturize them from the inside.

Then to salve our conscience we will eat a container of yogurt. But generally the yogurt is a fruit flavored kind, loaded with sugar that kills the friendly bacteria so beneficial to the colon.

Examine your own daily eating habits. How much of the food that you eat daily has been refined, processed, degraded, manipulated, machined, mauled or mangled and then cooked to death?

And how much of the food you eat daily is fresh, live and really nutritious? When was the last time you drank a 12 ounce glass of carrot juice? Or have you never had this exhilarating experience?

4

HOW JUICES RESTORE HEALTH NATURALLY

**Our Food
Is Not
Getting
Better**

Dr. Ross Hume Hall, head of the Department of Biochemistry at McMaster University, says:

> The food industry is trying to thwart natural processes in every way for its own convenience and profit. I've never seen any of these food people actually detail their argument that there would be world starvation without food additives.

And Jacqueline Verrett, a biochemist and researcher for the U.S. Food and Drug Administration, foresees a grim future for consumers. She remarks:

> This outlook for a bigger, better chemical feast might be described as a collective Last Supper, for we have virtually no idea of the cumulative effect on living tissue, especially after years of consumption.

I believe we are now seeing some of the results of our disastrous eating habits. And that is why it is doubly important that we discover in our own lives how live juices can restore our health . . . naturally and thus aid us in coping with the increasing day-to-day problems with which each of us is faced.

Surviving The Healing Crisis

A large number of individuals, even in affluent America, are starving to death on a full stomach! It is not the quantity that we eat that corrects a deficiency. One person has remarked that one-third of what we eat keeps us alive; the other two-thirds keeps the doctor alive.

In a majority of acute diseases we experience a healing crisis. This is the result of the body struggling to free itself from its load of toxic poisons. How often, instead of providing our body with live juices and help it release these poisons . . . we bottle them up by using drugs which can, in effect, be a stopper. We believe we are healed . . . only to be plagued in later years with the same or additional ailments.

Golden liquids of great healing power are released when raw juices are unlocked from the cells of plants. These vital liquids

Unlock
Healing
Power

can gently coax our body back to normal.
John B. Lust, a leader in raw juice therapy
says:

> . . . juices, subtle in their action, yet
> more potent than any medicine, and
> without the toxic effect of drugs, can
> eliminate or prevent many of the
> chronic and degenerative diseases
> with which human beings are af-
> flicted.[1]

4 Horsemen
of
Poor Health

There are 4 Horsemen of Poor Health:

1. Overeating
2. Not eating the right foods
3. Sedentary life
4. Sluggish metabolism

How many of these Horsemen are active
helping you race to an early grave?

Most Americans overeat and do not eat the
right foods. If we eat salads, we generally
reach for iceberg lettuce which just about
gets a nutritional ZERO. And we always
push aside the parsley on our plate. And
rarely, since the advent of the automobile,
do we exercise . . . except to get up and
change the TV dial. For many, probably
the most strenuous exercise they get is
simply getting up out of bed every morning.

You Can't
Fool
Mother Nature

All of these can contribute to a sluggish
metabolism. You can't fool Mother Nature.
Nor can you fool with your fuel and not
suffer the consequences. The 4 Horsemen
contribute to poor digestion and also to

---

[1] John B. Lust, *Raw Juice Therapy* (England: Thorsons Publishers, Ltd.), 1958, p. 1.

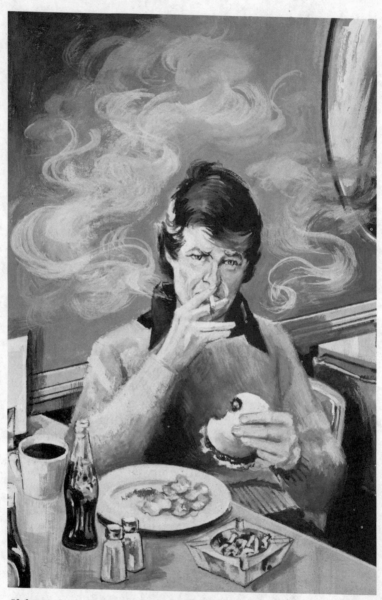

If these elements are typical of your dining habits, you should make sure to have adequate hospitalization insurance.

poor assimilation of food. Because of this, our cells start to degenerate and break down. Then the normal process of cell replacement and cell rebuilding slows down. Our body begins to grow old. And we find our resistance to disease starts to quickly diminish!

When the cells break down and die at a faster rate than new cells are built . . . aging begins to set in.

Live Cells Need Live Juices

Juices . . . live juices help quickly to eliminate the dead and dying cells while at the same time, speed up the building of new cells. And at the same time, all the toxic wastes that have interfered with the nourishment of the cells are eliminated. Our sluggish metabolic rate and our cell oxygenation are restored.

What is metabolism? Metabolism is the sum of all the physical and chemical changes that take place within an organism. It involves two processes: assimilation (or *building up*) and disintegration (or *tearing-down*). Thus it affects our life-giving energy and disposal of poisons toxic to our system.

Awaken a Sluggish Metabolism

The next time you meet a friend drawn, dragging and despondent who is puffing a cigarette, sipping on a cola while downing a hamburger between mouthfuls of french fries, chances are he has the slowest metabolism this side of El Paso.

And if he is drinking that beer that gives him *"gusto"* he will not only go around in this world . . . once . . . but he may go around very quickly!

But let's get back to cells. Every living thing is built of cells. That means your body is made up of countless millions of cells. Our life is based on a vast, continuous series of chemical changes that take place in and around our cells.

**Stop
Starving
Your Cells!**

To carry out its functions, each cell must obtain a constant supply of raw materials to work with. These raw materials — nutrients — come from the food we eat.

Every <u>minute</u>, it is estimated that some 300 million cells die in the body. In a healthy body, these are replaced quickly by the division of cells that remain. But when we do not get the proper nutrients into our body . . . we open the door to illness.

That's where raw, live juices come in. They are our life insurance to make sure our cells are happy and healthy! And believe me . . . it doesn't pay to get a cell angry at you! Every cell has a "memory bank." And angry cells never forget!

5

HOW FRUIT JUICES
CAN CLEANSE YOUR SYSTEM

**My Quality
of Life
Improved
100%**

Are you old enough to remember Nelson Eddy singing to Jeanette McDonald:

*Ah, sweet mystery of life
at last I've found you . . .*

That's what I wanted to sing when I discovered the life-giving forces of freshly prepared fruit and vegetable juices. My quality of living improved 100%

It is 10:15 on a Wednesday morning. And first thing I did this morning was drink 12 ounces of live juices. In my juice cocktail were the juices of a pear and an apple. I call my juice drink Life's Golden Glow and the ingredients appear elsewhere in this book.

**Raw Juice
Therapy
Is a
Valid Therapy**

Raw juice therapy is as much a valid therapy for illness as any medical therapy. It is simpler, less costly and can be far more effective. When God created the human body, he created the parts so that each one would function in harmony with all the other units of the body . . . if properly fueled.

When this "ease" turns into "dis-ease" it is a warning sign that the body units are not working in perfect harmony. Quite possibly the reason could be a lack of proper fuel. Raw juice therapy quickly provides that fuel.

It must be remembered that fresh fruit juices are the **cleansers** of the human system. And vegetable juices are the **builders** and the regenerators of the body.

Why Raw Juices Work Faster!

Within 15 minutes after drinking on an empty stomach ... raw juices begin to enter the bloodstream through the digestive processes. Now that's fast action! Only honey acts quicker!

While juices are absorbed by the blood stream quickly ... if you have an illness, don't expect miracles overnight. You should notice an improvement in vitality within a week or two. However, nature works slowly but efficiently. And many have discovered that stubborn physical ailments respond marvelously when one faithfully uses raw juice therapy over many months.

Make It A Daily Habit

Frankly, whether well or ill, I would recommend the drinking of live juices daily for your entire lifetime. It is nature's insurance for a healthy life.

Remember, raw fruit juices are the cleansers of the human body. And when the clean-up operation begins it is not uncommon for one to go through a "healing crisis." If you have lived on junk food, highly seasoned food, starches and candy, cola and cake . . . you can expect distress when starting a juice program. This does not mean that the raw juices do not agree with you. What it means is that the juices are not compatible with the unhealthy condition of your stomach or colon. Many mistake these irritating symptoms as an indication that the juices "*do not agree*" with them. On the contrary, the "*goodies*" (juices) are engaged in combat with the "*baddies*" junk food . . . and the ultimate outcome should be one where all the poisons are uprooted and booted out of your body.

During the course of this raw juice therapy you may experience eruptions, headaches, fevers and diarrhea. It is always wise to keep your doctor advised of any change you anticipate making in your diet.

Improving Circulation

Raw juices, particularly oranges and lemons, contain the greatest concentrations of bioflavonoids. Bioflavonoids have proven an effective treatment for problems of circulation.

Picture your body as a giant network of roads. The interstate highways are the **arteries and veins.** These are the largest tubes of the circulatory system. Arterties all carry blood **away** from the heart, and veins all carry blood **toward** the heart.

The state roads are the **arterioles.** They branch off from the artery into smaller vessels and supply blood to the skin, the muscles and other organs.

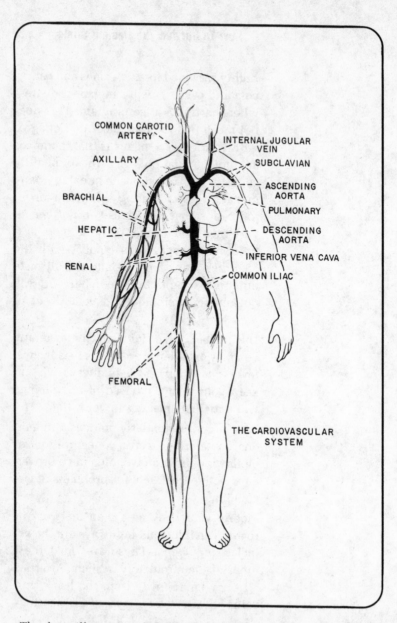

COMMON CAROTID
ARTERY

INTERNAL JUGULAR
VEIN

AXILLARY

SUBCLAVIAN

ASCENDING
AORTA

BRACHIAL

PULMONARY

HEPATIC

DESCENDING
AORTA

INFERIOR VENA CAVA

RENAL

COMMON ILIAC

FEMORAL

THE CARDIOVASCULAR
SYSTEM

The above illustration shows the cariovascular system of arteries and
veins. One must remember, however, that your body is made up of a
vast network of some 60,000 miles of tubing which carries blood to
every part of your body. When these tubes become narrow or clogged,
serious illness occurs. Live juices, taken daily, can play a major role
in keeping these tubes healthy and free-flowing.

The country roads are the minute **capillaries.** They are branches which emerge from the **arterioles** *(state roads).* The capillaries average only one twenty-fifth of an inch in length, and a hundredth of that in diameter. The capillary wall is only one cell thick! Through this wall materials pass into and out of the blood.

Now all these roads . . . the arteries, the veins, the arterioles, the capillaries . . . represent the vast network of blood-carrying vessels. They penetrate every corner of the body, fueling, servicing and bathing with fluid every cell in every tissue. If all these circulation tubes were unraveled, the total length would be many thousands of miles. Is it any wonder that the life is in the blood *(Leviticus 17:11)?*

You Are As Old As Your Blood Vessels

A man is as old as his blood vessels. Many people with arthritis suffer from fragile capillaries. Elderly people often become victims of atherosclerosis. In this blood vessel disease the vessel walls lose their elasticity as the walls become thick and less flexible. As it further progresses nutrients fail to get through because of these road blocks.

Now can you see why it is important to daily include live fruit juices in your diet. They are assimilated within 15 minutes . . . get right to work in your body . . . providing not only bioflavonoids but also a host of minerals and vitamins to keep the highways of your body (the blood vessels) feeding and nourishing your entire system.

Strengthen Your Heart Naturally

Live fruit juices, whose nourishment will reach every part of your body, will be a great aid in also strengthening your heart action and kidney functioning.

Now be honest with yourself. Look at a hamburger. Walk around a french fry. And examine the cola (and uncola) drinks that promise you a new world. And ask yourself the question: Why load up your highway of blood vessels with junk cars when you can have sleek, fast-moving apples with pear horsepower and orange wheels and a lemon top!

6

HOW VEGETABLE JUICES
CAN REGENERATE A TIRED, WORN-OUT BODY

Someone In Your Army Is Sleeping

Your body is an army. And if you are sick it is evident that some of the troops are sleeping while others are goldbricking. Is it any wonder? What did you feed the army this morning . . . or last night?

Fried eggs and bacon for breakfast? No wonder your army is asleep! It's time to give them live juices. For juices, live juices, provide concentrated instant power.

In the previous chapter we told you that fresh fruit juices are the cleansers of the human system. And because fresh fruit juices are stimulating, it is best to take fruit juice drinks before 2 PM in the day. (Otherwise, you may have trouble sleeping.)

Why Not Eat The Whole Vegetable?

While fruit juices <u>clean</u> your system, <u>vegetable juices are the builders</u> or regenerators of the human body.

You may ask:

> Why not eat the WHOLE vegetables and fruits, instead of extracting the juice?

A good question. But the answer is simple. It would require many hours of digestive activity for you to eat solid food before its nourishment is finally available to your body cells and tissues.

Now we are not advocating, by any means, that you should discontinue eating solid foods. What we are suggesting is that at least twice a day you should supplement your diet with fresh, live vegetable and fruit juices.

Juices Get To Work Fast!

Juices are quickly digested, assimilated within a matter of minutes with a minimum of exertion on the part of your digestive system! This enables you to get volume nourishment within 15 minutes without the laborious chewing on some 10 carrots, an apple, a pear and stalks of celery ... as an example.

Vegetable juices contain all the vitamins, all the minerals, all the amino acids, all the enzymes and salts needed by the human body. They must be juiced fresh and in their raw state, however.

With a proper juicer, the fibers of the fruit or vegetable are triturated; that means, the cells of the fibers are ripped open so the full benefits of the vitamins, enzymes and other nutrients are converted to juice. Not all juicers on the market give this action. You might ask:

**How Much
Juice
Should I
Drink Daily?**

> How much juice should one drink daily?

The answer is, basically, as much as you can comfortably assimilate.

Most nutritionists agree that the minimum daily juice intake should be at least one pint (16 ounces). However better results are experienced when two to six pints are taken daily. I used to drink one pint daily but then began also drinking another pint about 3 every afternoon. I found this additional juice made a world of difference in my overall well-being. The more juice we drink the quicker will be the results.

What are some of the basic vegetable juices that are builders and regenerators of our body?

**The Basic
Juice Builders
Of Our Body**

Carrot juice is nature's beauty treatment! It is effective for colitis, ulcers, circulation and is a guardian angel of the nervous system. Its qualities are many. There is more protein in one 8 ounce glass of carrot juice than there is in an egg!

One glass of carrot juice will supply us with iron equivalent to what we would get in two ounces of calves' liver.

One glass of carrot juice can provide half the recommended daily amount of calcium! (And more riboflavin than a cup of

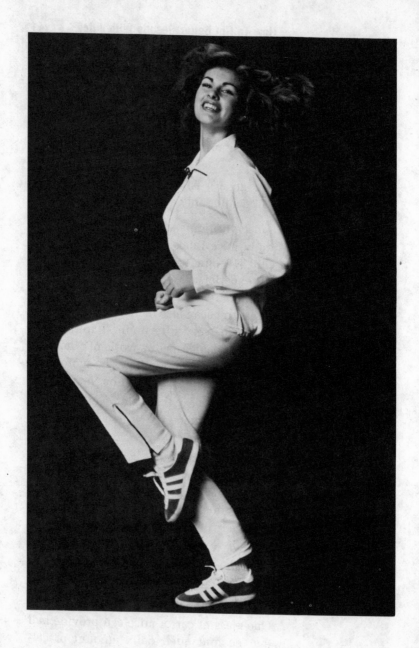

Live juices can put a new spring in your step!

milk).

You may be surprised to learn that raw carrot juice can be combined with milk without curdling and is an excellent juice for babies.

Celery juice is a giant source of magnesium, sodium and iron. Celery is nature's nerve tonic. I juice at least 8-10 stalks a day. And although my days abound in stress, I find that the celery juice keeps me calm and worry-free. Celery also is an excellent aid *(in juice form)* for a sound sleep.

Cabbage juice contains sulphur and chlorine and these are excellent properties in cleaning the mucous membrane of the stomach and the intestinal tract. Many have found raw cabbage juice beneficial in reducing weight and for stomach ulcers. Because cabbage juice is powerful, one should start off with 2 or 3 ounces initially, until your system becomes acclimated to the juice. It is important to remember never to change your diet drastically overnight. Ease into a new diet and the results will be more palatable for you in this change-over period.

Tips On Preparing Food Nutritionally

While writing this book . . . as a re-vitalizer . . . I drink 4 ounces of cranberry juice and water combined, every one-half hour. I find such a practice gives me consistent energy and supplies my body with the necessary liquids.

Peeling or scraping vegetables will remove a great deal of the vitamins and minerals. Soaking vegetables in water will cause the vegetable to lose much of its value as water acts as a leech.

We cook too many of our vegetables. Cooking or canning or preserving robs vegetables of a large amount of the mineral and vitamin content.

Juices That Help Teenagers

Vegetable juices are beneficial for teenagers as well and contribute greatly to the normal development of glands and helps avoids many of the pimply conditions so usual during this period.

Those who are ill and cannot tolerate raw vegetables or much food will welcome raw vegetable juice drinks as a nourishing revitalizer and builder of the human body.

7

HOW TO BE YOUNG AGAIN!

Freshness
Is
The Key

With the food we eat these days it's a wonder we are still alive!

This reminds me of the bachelor who was eating breakfast in a restaurant when he saw the following note written on an egg:

> Should this meet the eye of some young man who desires to marry a farmer's daughter, age 19, write . . . . .

The bachelor wrote and in a few days received the following note:

> Your letter came too late. I am now married and have four children!

It is obvious we cannot hope to be young again eating food that is aged, injected, devitalized, extruded, additive-added and has been fried and then has died!

Now they have developed milk that will not go bad, even if not kept in the refrigerator; and it can be stored on a shelf indefinitely. Can you imagine where all the vitality and nutrients have gone? They have long since been buried! No wonder we reach middle age quickly!

Middle age is when your age starts to show around your middle. Middle age is that time when one is always thinking that in a week or two he will feel just as good as ever.

The Perils of Middle Age

One diplomatic individual remarked:

> There are three ages of man —
> Youth, age and
> "you are looking wonderful."

If you are reading this book, chances are that you are over 50 and you have been told

<u>verbally</u>

> You are looking wonderful

<u>and silently</u>

FOR YOUR AGE!

When The Spring of Your Life Turns to Fall

Middle age is later than you think . . . and sooner than you expect. That's what I discovered when I hit 50 on November 12, 1975. I was soon reminded that

> My get up and go . . .
> Got up and went!

I realized that life is a stream which drifts flowers in spring but blocks of ice in winter. And it appeared to me that the springtime of my life was shifting into fall with winter looming on the horizon.

Aches, pains, fatigue, sleepless nights, faint mysterious ailments all were warning signs that winter's wintry blasts were turning spring streams into a sluggish waterway.

Life can only be understood backwards; but it must be lived forwards. And although I could reflect back on the vibrancy of my youth, its carefree days, its bubbling bouyancy of good health . . . my life would plod ahead through the 50's and on into the 60's . . . and if 50 felt this bad . . . how much worse would 51 be?

I mentioned in chapter 1 how I discovered the benefits of sound nutrition and the daily drinking of live juices. And when I discovered this, I discovered the secret of becoming young again . . . not numerically, of course; but young in spirit, in vitality, in direction and in zestful purpose!

Never . . . For A Million Dollars

And never . . . not for a million dollars would I trade this for a daily meal of fried eggs, bacon, pancakes, hamburgers, french fries, shrimp, lobster, cola drinks or a host of other junk foods that are dead and help the dying die quicker!

You must remember, for 50 years I was eating basically an incorrect diet . . . one consisting mainly of cooked, devitalized foods.

I Saw Immediate Results

When I changed my diet to live foods and live juices, I saw immediate results. But it took 1½ years to achieve what I believe is the top rung of the vibrant living ladder. This time was spent in draining the body of its poisons and giving the cells a new lease on life.

I tried various juice drink combinations and only after several months did I discover what worked best for me. Now everyone's body is different and what is best for me may not be necessarily the most beneficial for you. But I pass this information on as background.

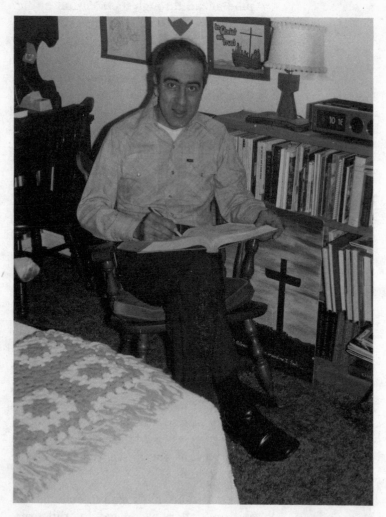

Spiritual food is as important as sound, nutritional food. Every morning, before breakfast, I sit in a rocking chair and quietly read and meditate upon a chapter from the Bible. Then I kneel at the bed and pray asking God to guide me through the day. If you don't follow this practice, you are missing the greatest key to a happy, healthy life. Why not start tomorrow morning?

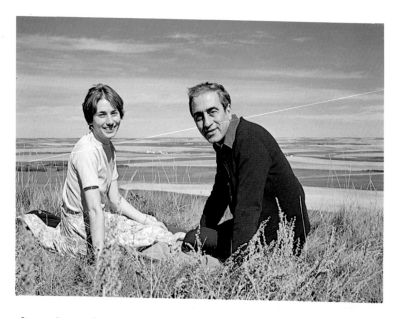

It was September 2, 1978! Our daughter, Diane, and I sat on top of one of the hills in Three Hills, Alberta, Canada. Both of us have discovered how live juices can restore health . . . naturally. What a joy it was that day to drink in God's handiwork in a panorama of nature, unspoiled by man's "progress."

IMPORTANT

This book was primarily written to introduce those in the healing arts the valid concept of raw juice therapy.

Nothing in this book is intended to constitute medical treatment or advice of any nature.

Moreover, it is recommended that before any change in diet is made, one should visit his doctor for initial and continued supervision.

The raw juice combinations on the following pages are a compilation of data reported for information purposes only. By publishing them, we do **not** imply that they will cure any disease.

JUICES THAT SHOULD NOT BE USED ALONE

The following juices should **not** be used alone. They should always be used in combination with other juices.

Asparagus
Beet
Beet greens
Dandelion
Garlic

Lemon
Parsley
Spinach
Turnip

HINTS ON MAKING LIVE JUICE DRINKS

For full nutrient value . . .
juices
should be made fresh
and consumed immediately.
Do not make a juice drink and then let it sit or place in a refrigerator and drink later.

Make the juice at the time you are ready to drink it.

When preparing fruits and vegetables to juice . . . remember these hints for top mineral and vitamin value:

1. **DEEP COLOR BEST**
   If the vegetable is green, the deeper green it is, the higher the mineral value. Avoid iceberg lettuce and blanched celery, as an example.

   A deep red or deep yellow apple generally indicates a higher mineral content, etc.

2. **THE SWEETER THE BETTER**
   The sweeter tasting the carrot, the better. It indicates it has been grown in organically rich soil and the carrot is rich in mineral and vitamin content.

   If you bite into a stalk of celery and find it bitter, don't buy it. It has been grown in mineral-poor soil.

3. **DRINK SUFFICIENT JUICE DAILY**
   Drinking only 6-8 ounces of live juices daily will not prove very beneficial. Nutritionists have found that optimum benefit comes from drinking 16 ounces of juice twice a day . . . once in early morning and once in mid-afternoon. For those with terminal or extremely hazardous diseases, some nutritionists suggest drinking 16 ounces 4-8 times a day. [1]

4. **CHECK WITH YOUR DOCTOR**
   NEVER change your diet without first consulting with your doctor.

---

[1] Gary & Steve Null, The Complete Handbook of Nutrition (New York: Dell Publishing Co., Inc.), 1972, p. 194.

CARROT JUICE

Nutritionists recommend for:

Cancers
Digestive Disturbances of Infants
Dry Skin, Dermatitis, Acne
Infections of Eyes, Throat (Tonsils, Sinuses)
Intestinal ailments
Nursing Mothers
Sterility
Ulcers
Urinary infections

Background Information

Carrots are richest in Vitamin A and Potassium. One 10-ounce cup averages 12,000 units of Vitamin A. One pint of carrot juice daily, has more constructive body value than 25 pounds of calcium tablets (N. W. Walker, D. Sci.). Carrots also contain a good supply of: magnesium, iron, and phosphorus.

Carrot soup for treating digestive disturbances of infants has been favored by Drs. J. Stroder and W. Scholtz of the University of Wurzburg, Germany. Carrot soup has been used with excellent results for treating infantile diarrhea in tests with 450 cases.

The soup is prepared as follows: 16 ounces of fresh carrots cooked in 5 ounces of water in a pressure cooker for 15 minutes. The pulp is sieved and diluted with hot water up to 1 quart. A pinch of salt is added. The soup is given in as large amounts as possible. After 24 hours, milk is given and thereafter the amount of milk is gradually increased and the amount of soup decreased. (Source: Nutrition Abstracts and Reviews, Dr. P. Selander, Kristianstad Hospital, Malmo, Sweden)

In another study with infants it was concluded that 3 to 8 month old children on the basis of smell and taste prefer carrots to tomatoes, peas, beans or mixed vegetables.

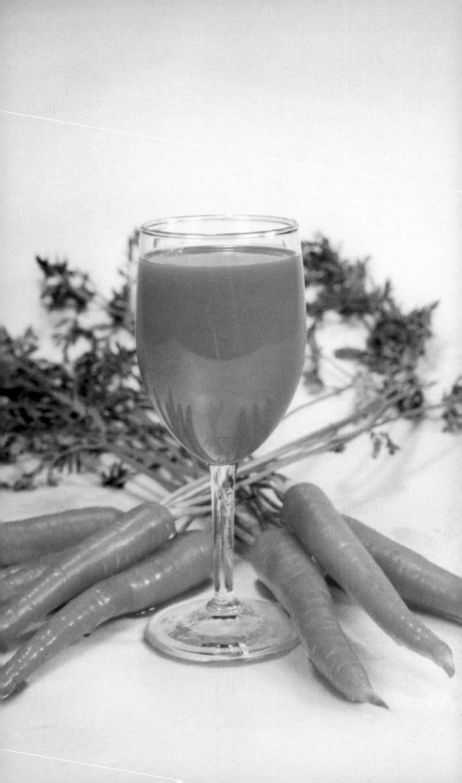

CELERY JUICE

Nutritionists recommend for:

Arthritis
Asthma
Bronchial and Lung Troubles
Diuretic (water removing)
Hemorrhoids
Insomnia
Nervous Tension
Neurasthenia
  (a type of neurosis, usually the result of emotional conflicts, charac-
  terized by irritability, fatigue, weakness, anxiety)
Tobacco Users
Weight Reduction

Background Information

Celery juice in hot weather is a soothing and comforting drink and has
the effect of normalizing the body temperature (while others may be
drenched in perspiration and sweltering).

Celery is highest in potassium, sodium, calcium and phosphorus and
very high in magnesium and iron content. It is invaluable as a food
for the blood cells.

Celery juice has more than four times as much **organic** sodium as it
does calcium. This is beneficial to those whose diet has been high in
concentrated sugars, starches . . . such as bread, cakes, cereals, dough-
nuts, spaghetti or any food with flour. Do not confuse **organic** sodium
found in celery juice with the insoluble, inorganic elements found in
table salt. Hardening of the arteries and varicose veins may result in
excessive use of table salt. Nutritionists believe it is best to get your
salt through **organic** sodium found in celery juice.

Eating celery sticks between meals quells hunger pains and thus
achieves moderate, consistent weight reduction. (A study made by
Dr. Clarence Bernstein and Dr. S. K. Klotz in Florida)

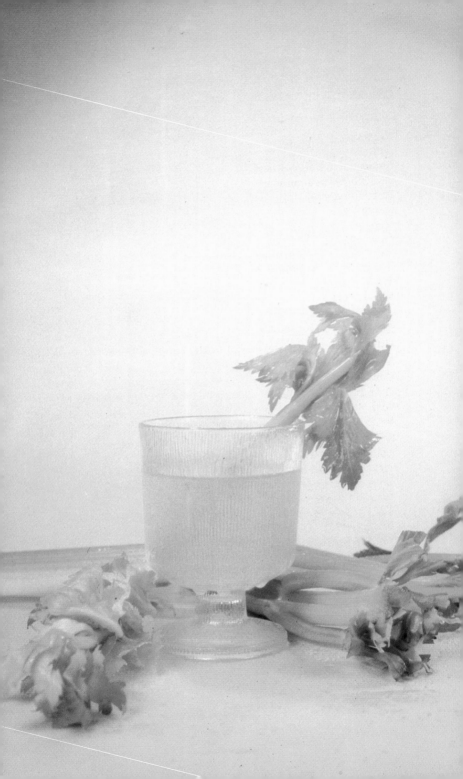

CARROT/CELERY/PARSLEY Juice

Nutritionists recommend for:

Kidneys
Optic Nerves
Sympathetic Nerve System
> *(A part of the nervous system which is concerned with control of involuntary bodily functions; that is, glands, muscle tissue and the heart)*

Juice Combination

Carrot	8 ounces
Celery	6 ounces
Parsley	2 ounces

Background Information

Parsley is very high in vitamin C and also has substantial amounts of calcium, magnesium, phosphorus, potassium and vitamin A.

Parsley is an excellent digestive aid. At my back door, I maintain a parsley bed in a cold frame. This supplies me with parsley throughout the year. With my salad I try to include a handful of parsley daily (4-5 sprigs). When dining in a restaurant with friends I grab their parsley off their plate (since they don't eat it anyway) and I feel healthier for it.

My favorite salad is a Lebanese salad my mother taught me, called *Tabbouleh*. I renamed it **"Salem's Salad."** The recipe is found in the book, How To Eat Your Way Back to Vibrant Health.[1] The basic ingredient of this salad is parsley.

Caution

Concentrated parsley juice should never be taken alone in quantities greater than one tablespoon at a time. It is very potent. If taken by itself in excess, it will overstimulate the nervous system.

---

[1] Salem Kirban, How To Eat Your Way Back To Vibrant Health, Kent Road, Huntingdon Valley, Penna. 19006. (Send $3.95 plus 50¢ for postage)

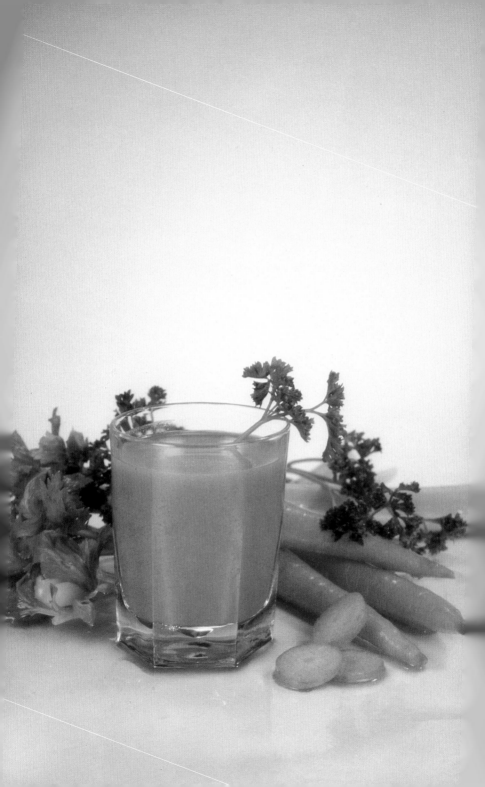

CARROT/CELERY Juice

Nutritionists recommend for:
Arthritis
Insomnia
*Multiple Sclerosis
Nervous Tension
*Parkinson's Disease

Juice Combination

Carrot   8 ounces
Celery   8 ounces
(Include celery tops in juicing)

Background Information

* Multiple Sclerosis is a hardening within the nervous system resulting from degeneration of nervous elements, as in the <u>myelin</u> sheath.
Myelin is composed of cholesterol and fatty acids. A fatlike substance
forms the principal component of the myelin sheath of nerve fibers.
There is no specific medical treatment for this disease.

* Parkinson's Disease is an organic disease of the brain associated
with tremors and muscle rigidity. Chronic constipation is associated
with this disease. A main cause is Arteriosclerosis of the blood vessels
in the brain; commonly known as *"hardening of the arteries."*

Sound nutritional practices are important for those in good health and
extremely vital to those in ill health. However, nothing in this book or
on this page should imply that by drinking a juice combination your
health problems will disappear.

An excellent series of articles on Multiple Sclerosis appeared in the
June, July, August issues of LET'S LIVE magazine in 1978.[1]

---

[1] Let's Live, 444 North Larchmont Blvd., Los Angeles, California 90004,
(213) 469-3901.

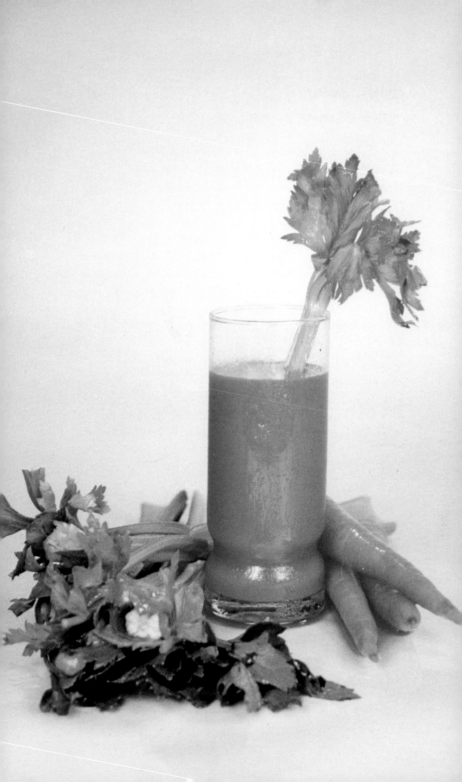

CELERY/CABBAGE Juice

Nutritionists recommend for:

Constipation
Skin Problems
Ulcers

Juice Combination

| Celery | 3 ounces |
| Cabbage | 3 ounces |

* *(Five times a day in 6-ounce quantities)*

Background Information

* Cabbage juice is strong and initially should be sipped slowly in small quantity. One who is ill may experience gas and digestive upset initially. Dr. Garnett Cheney of Stanford University School of Medicine treated ulcer patients with cabbage juice therapy ... giving his patients six-ounce quantities five times a day. Fresh cabbage juice *(vitamin U)* proved therapeutic.

When raw carrot juice *(10 ounces)* is added to the juice combination above, the vitamin C becomes a cleansing agent and has been helpful for those suffering infection of the gums *(pyorrhea)*.

Do not cook the cabbage nor add salt to it. These destroy the nutritive values.

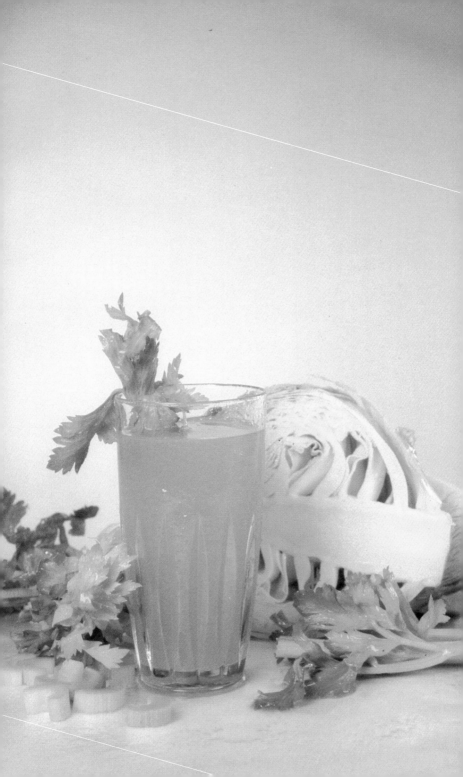

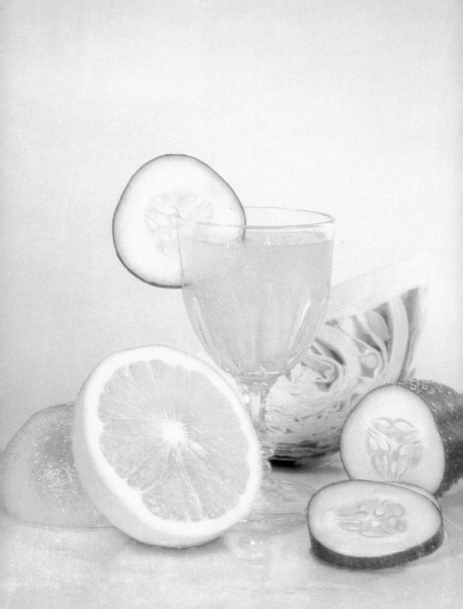

CABBAGE/CUCUMBER/GRAPEFRUIT Juice

Nutritionists recommend for:

Antiseptic
Digestive Disturbances
Diuretic
*Intestinal Cleansing

Juice Combination

Cabbage	6 ounces
Cucumber	6 ounces
Grapefruit	4 ounces

Background Information

* This juice combination should **not** be taken in cases of colitis.

Cucumber juice is probably the best natural diuretic known. Its high chlorine and sulphur properties make it excellent for cleansing the mucous membranes of both the stomach and intestinal tract. Cucumbers are also high in potassium. As a diuretic, it can be taken by itself. Grapefruit juice is also high in potassium. Many hypoglycemics who cannot tolerate orange juice can drink grapefruit juice.

SALEM'S
Velvety, Verdant, Versatile,
Virtuous, Venturous, Vivacious Victory JUICE

Nutritionists recommend for:

(They never heard of it!)

Salem Kirban uses it for:

A general, all purpose, vibrant energy drink

* Juice Combination

Carrot (3-4)	4 ounces
Celery (4 stalks)	4 ounces
Pear (1)	4 ounces
Apple (1)	4 ounces
Lecithin	2 Tablespoons (granular type)

* Ounces are approximate.

Background Information

I make no claims for this juice combination. I have found it has revolutionized my total health picture. At this writing, 1978, I am 52½. I have been drinking this combination of 16 ounces twice a day (9 AM and 2:30 PM) for the last two years. I awake alert, alive and full of energy. Rarely do I experience fatigue. Empirically speaking, I feel great.[1] I feel better now at 52 than I did at 17!

I include a pear in my juice drink because the minerals are beneficial to the prostate. I include an apple because the pectin in the apple is beneficial for the heart. I take the lecithin because I personally believe it is good both for the heart and the nerves. This juice combination works wonders for me. This is to no way imply, however, that it will do anything for you. It's my Victory Juice. And I love it. I am getting younger every day. I may even go back to high school!

---

[1] Doctors do not accept empirical evidence. Empirical means: *relying solely on observation and practical experience without reference to scientific principles.* While I believe in scientific principles, I do not let them get in my way in drinking live juices such as **SALEM'S 7 V Juice.** I believe **live bodies** are nourished by **live juices** and **live foods.**

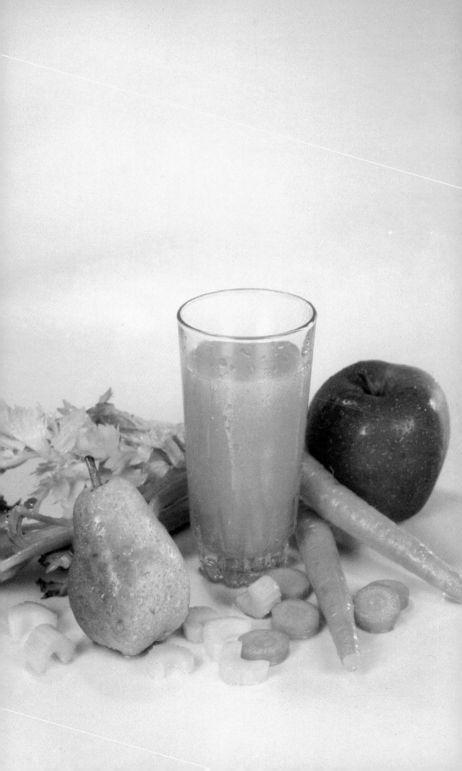

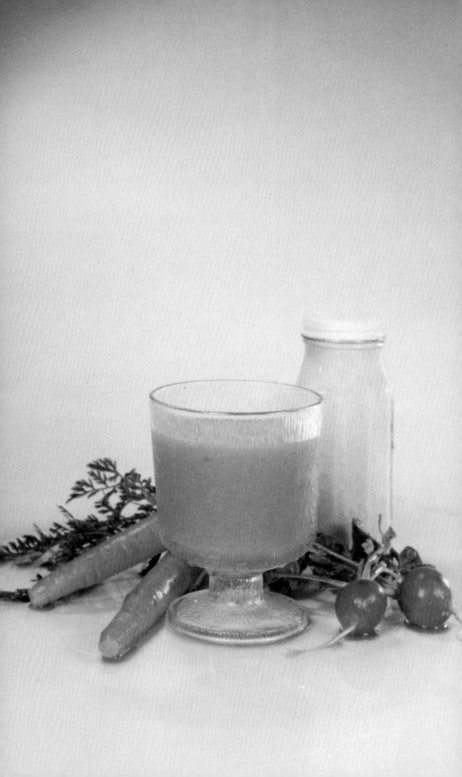

CARROT/RADISH/HORSERADISH Juice

Nutritionists recommend for:

Diuretic
*Dropsy
Sinus Trouble

Juice Combination

John B. Lust suggests:
One-half teaspoonful of fresh horseradish should be taken twice a day between meals . . . it must be kept cold and moistened with plenty of lemon juice. Never add vinegar. White distilled vinegar and wine vinegar destroy the tissues of the membranes lining the stomach and intestines. Do not mix anything else besides lemon juice to the horseradish . . . This will at first cause a sensation in the head which will create copious tears. This should be continued for weeks or months, until the horseradish sauce can be eaten without any sensation resulting from it.[1]

Carrot   14 ounces
Radish   2 ounces
    (including radish tops)

Background Information

* Dropsy is a condition rather than a disease. It occurs most in people over sixty and is an accumulation of fluid in the tissues and cavities. It often is an indication that the heart is not functioning efficiently.

Nutritionists believe the above juice combination is a natural cleanser of the abnormal mucous in the system and that it effectively dissolves this mucous without damage to the membranes. Mucous is the result of eating concentrated starches (bread, cereal, etc.) and drinking too much milk.

Radish juice should never be taken alone or by those suffering from arthritis, gall stones, kidney stones or skin problems.

---

[1] John B. Lust, Raw Juice Therapy (England: Thorsons Publishers, Ltd.), 1959, pp. 68, 69.

CARROT/CUCUMBER/BEET Juice

Nutritionists recommend for:

Anemia
Fatigue
Gallstones
Kidney Stones
Low Blood Pressure
Menopause
Menstrual Disturbances
Sex Glands

Juice Combination

Carrot   6 ounces
Cucumber   5 ounces
Beet   5 ounces

(Include a few beet tops)

Background Information

While the quantity of iron in red beets is not high, it has been found that it is of a quality that furnishes excellent food for the red corpuscles of the blood. It tones the blood and acts as a cleansing agent.

Beet juice by itself *(2 or 3 ounces)* two or three times a day has been helpful to some women with menstrual disturbances. Many believe it is also very beneficial during menopause.

The juice combination of carrot, cucumber and beet furnish a high concentrate of minerals and is one of the best builders of the blood cells. These juices provide water soluble calcium so necessary for the human body.

Many have found this a rejuvenating and invigorating drink. Beets are high in potassium and beet greens are high not only in potassium but also in calcium, iron and vitamin A.

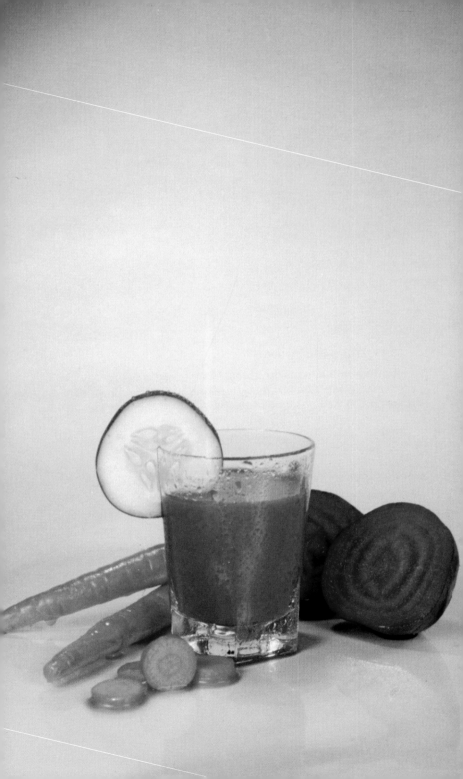

CARROT/APPLE Juice

Nutritionists recommend for:

Anemia
Arthritis
Complexion Problems
Constipation
Cystitis
Digestive Problems
Heart Trouble
Neuritis
Sluggish Gall Bladder
Tonic Rejuvenator

Juice Combination

Carrot	8 ounces
Apple	8 ounces

Background Information

Apples are a good body alkalizer. Apples were used successfully in Russia in experimental diets to relieve high blood pressure. Apples are low in sodium and therefore suitable for use in low sodium diets. Apples contain cellulose which provides needed bulk.

Apples also contain **pectin.** Experiments have shown that pectin has an anti-cholesterol effect if the quantity of pectin is sufficient. Pectin is credited also with detoxifying properties and surrounds viruses and thus reduces their motility (movement). Apples have a highly desireable cleansing effect on the teeth.

Scraped apple has been extensively used in Europe to treat infant intestinal disorders such as diarrhea and dysentery. Apples are high in potassium and phosphorus.

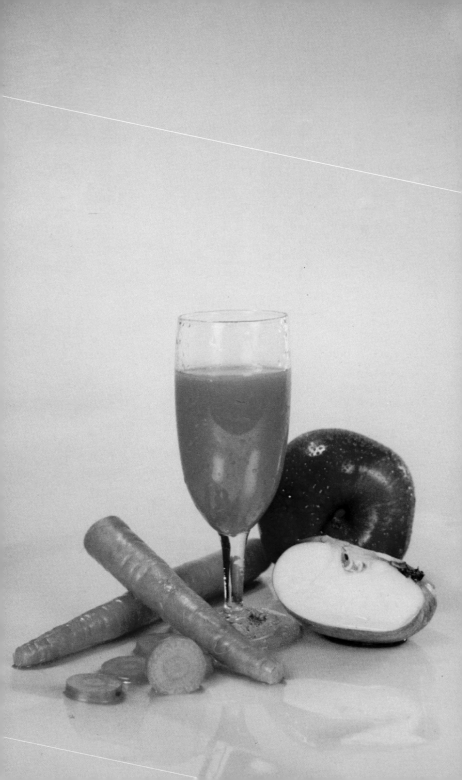

LETTUCE Juice

(Endive, Romaine, Crisphead or Iceberg)

Nutritionists recommend for:

Arteriosclerosis
Asthma
Digestive Disturbances
Fertility
*Hair Growth
Insomnia
Nervous Tension
Optic Nerves (Vision)

Juice Combination

Endive	4 ounces
Carrot	4 ounces
Celery	4 ounces
Spinach	4 ounces

Or

Lettuce	9 ounces
Spinach	6 ounces
Parsley	1 ounce

Background Information

* Much hair loss is caused by your genetic inheritance. If hair loss is due to poor nutrition habits; switching to sound nutrition practices may bring rewarding results.

For insomnia, drinking lettuce juice by itself *(crisphead)* may prove beneficial.

The Latin root word for lettuce is *"milk."* Lettuce *(crisphead, butter-head, cos or romaine and endive)* is high in both potassium and vitamin A.

Endive is popular with many who experience poor vision.

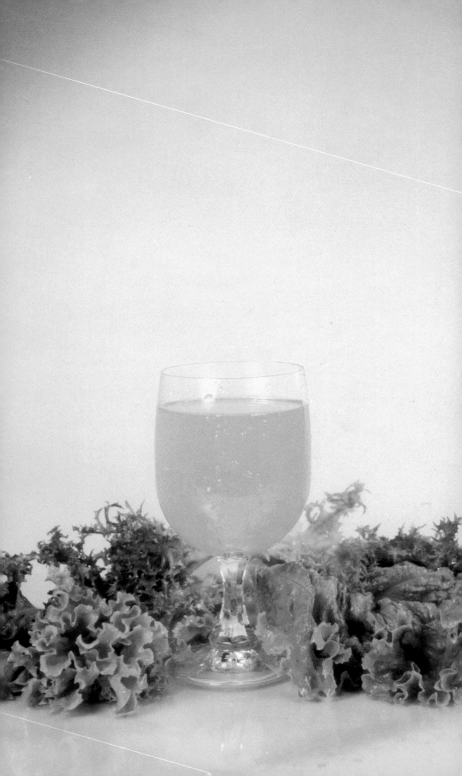

BLUEBERRY/HUCKLEBERRY Juice

Nutritionists recommend for:

Acidosis
*Diabetes
Dysentery
High Blood Pressure
Menstrual Disorders
Obesity

Juice Combination

| Blueberry | 8 ounces |
| Huckleberry | 8 ounces |

Background Information

This combination is known as a natural astringent, antiseptic and blood purifier. Russian women still use blueberries when one of the family has stomach trouble. Blueberries are richest in potassium.

Blueberries by 1670 were called huckleberries, although the huckleberry is of a different genus (species). Finally, in Scotland, the blackish blue berry was given the name blueberry. The American Indians found these berries highly beneficial.

* Diabetics, in particular, should consult with their doctor before making any change in diet.

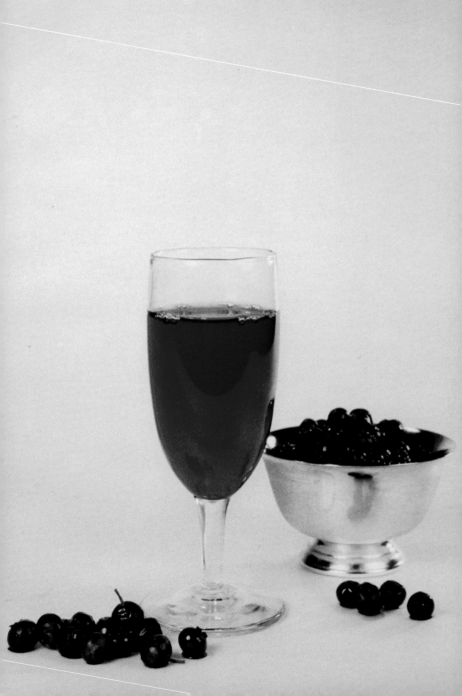

APPLE/BEET/CARROT/CELERY/SPINACH Juice

Nutritionists recommend for:

Acne
Allergies
Anemia
Angina
Arteriosclerosis
Constipation
Gallstones
Headaches
Hemorrhoids
Low Blood Pressure
Migraine

Juice Combination

Apple	4 ounces
Beet	2 ounces
Carrot	4 ounces
Celery	4 ounces
Spinach	2 ounces

Background Information

This food combination encompasses practically the entire range of organic minerals and salts. These foods are rich in potassium. If beet tops are used in juicing, you get the added benefit of iron. Beet tops and spinach should be used sparingly and not in excess. Those who suffer from <u>oxaluria</u> *(calcium crystals in urine)* or have a history of kidney stones, should avoid spinach, potatoes, beets, endive, tomatoes, dried figs, strawberries, plums, chocolate and tea.

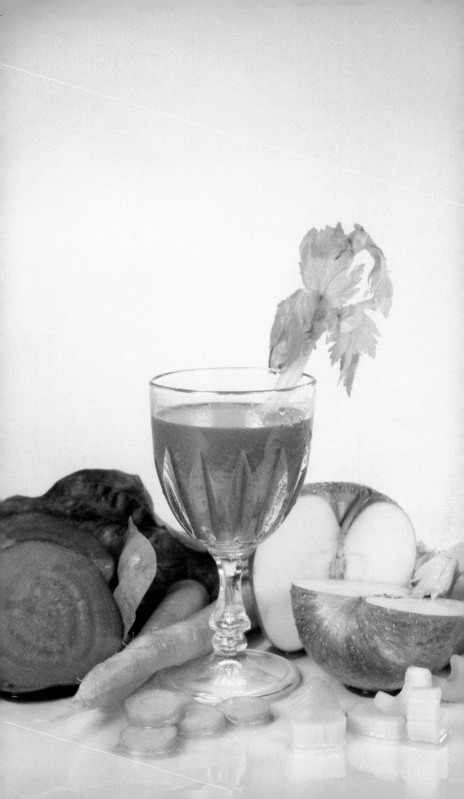

GREEN DRINK
Apple/Beet Tops/Celery/Comfrey/Endive/Green Beans/Okra

Nutritionists recommend for:

> Those
> whose sugar level
> is 5.50 or higher

Juice Combination

Beet Tops	About 4 tops
Celery	2 ounces
Endive	1 ounce
Green Beans	2 ounces
Comfrey Leaves	About 4 leaves
Okra	1 ounce
Apple	1 ounce

Background Information

Green Drink is best taken at mid-morning.

If 50-125 pounds .... drink 4 ounces
If 126-165 pounds .... drink 6 ounces
If 166 pounds or over .... drink 8 ounces

It should be consumed immediately after making to acquire full benefits from these nutrients.

Green drinks are an effective blood cleanser and blood builder. Green drink contains chlorophyll (an oxygen-producing agent) that is effective in combatting disease. Leafy vegetables can be put first into a blender with some water (about 2 cups) and then strained through a stainless steel sieve. For the celery, it is best to use the celery tops. The Juice Combination amounts given above are approximates and are not critical.

Other green, leafy vegetables can be substituted such as watercress, dandelion greens, turnip tops, garden pea leaves, romaine lettuce, mint and escarole.

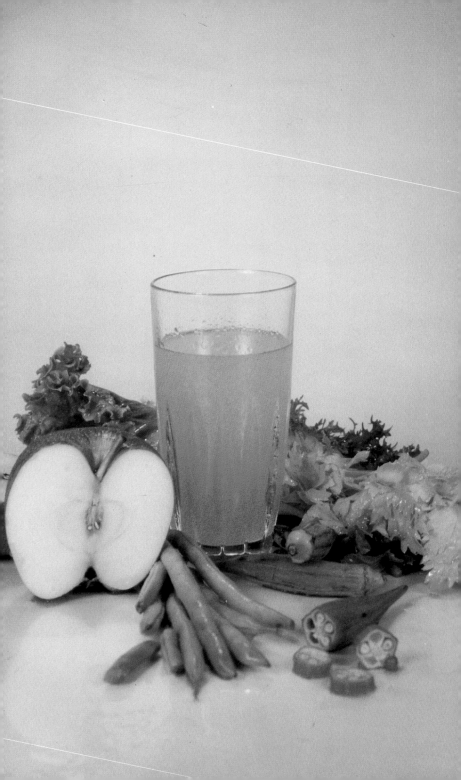

Hi there!

I wish you could have had lunch with me today!

My wife, Mary, made me one of my favorite dishes . . . a succulent combination of fresh sweet and hot peppers. It is our special day, our 32nd wedding anniversary.

And I am writing this on that day, August 17, 1978. I am typing this on the enclosed patio. The sun is shining. I can look out the window and see my garden (I turned part of my back lawn into a garden). The tomatoes are in full fruit as is the eggplant. The broccoli and brussel sprouts are coming along and soon the Okra will be ready!

For lunch we included a fresh tomato, plenty of peppers and I brought in a handful of fresh parsley from my parsley bed. It was delicious!

Finished lunch at 1 PM and then leisurely peddled my bicycle around the block a couple of times to get fresh air, exercise and Vitamin D.

One secret to good health is knowing how to <u>RELAX</u> after a meal. Now, I'm back again typing this last chapter.

The key to good health is found in the perfect blend of <u>body</u> *(world-consciousness)*, <u>soul</u> *(self-conscious life)* and <u>spirit</u> *(God-consciousness)*.

You could follow the best advice medical doctors have to offer, you could take the most recent drugs man has developed, you could drink all the fresh juice combinations possible . . . and still have poor health if your "whole being" attitude is negative. Negative emotions can produce a stagnant pool in your body. A happy, positive balance of Spirit, Soul and Body can provide a gentle flowing river.

Realign your priorities in life. If all you are concerned with is making money, holding down two jobs, to gain material possessions . . . you have missed life's true purpose.

Vibrant health begins with a happy heart.

> *A joyful heart is good medicine,*
> *But a broken spirit dries up the bones.*
> (Proverbs 17:22)

The choice is yours!

**My Recipe
For That
Golden Glow**

Here is my personal formula for that GOLDEN GLOW:

Every morning, upon arising, I juice in a juicer:

4-6 carrots
4   stalks of celery
1   apple
1   pear

This makes about 1 tall glass (16 ounces) of live juice. To this I add:

2 tablespoons of Lecithin granules

Many nutritionists believe the pear supplies valuable minerals to the prostate and assure a healthy gland. I have found that lecithin helps me eliminate nervous tension.

Every afternoon at 3 PM, I juice:

4-6 carrots
6   stalks of celery
    and add
2   tablespoons of Lecithin granules

And in the evening, before retiring I drink

4 ounces of distilled water with 2 tablespoons of Lecithin granules

I can't promise you that you will be a teenager again ... but you may have more energy and vibrancy than today's youngsters!

8

HOW TO REGAIN
THAT SCHOOLGIRL COMPLEXION

**How To Delay
The Ravages
Of Time**

A woman deserves no credit for her beauty at sixteen . . . but beauty at age 60 is her own soul's doing!

And the best thing to save for your old age is YOURSELF. Most women not only respect old age, they approach it with extreme caution. The longest period in a woman's life is the 10 years between the time she is 39 and 40.

For it is here that the ravages of time soon start to give evidence of age. And that evidence often first appears on our skin.

Is it any wonder that the cosmetic industry has a bonanza of profits. The poorer we eat . . . the bigger their business . . . for by outward application of lotions and creams we try to renew youthful skin, supple and blemish-free. But the answer is not what we put on the outside that counts . . . but what goes inside our body that makes the difference! And here is where juices play a major role in helping us restore that youthful complexion.

**Be Kind
To Your Skin**

Many people think of skin as just something needed to hold one's body together. But our skin is actually an organ of the body. It is the largest of the body organs. In an adult the total skin area is more than 18½ square feet and weighs about six pounds! This is almost double the weight of the brain.

**Your
First Line
Of Defense**

Skin is our first line of defense against invasion by bacteria, viruses and parasites. It is an agent of secretion and excretion and is a regulator of body temperature.

Each square inch of skin has 78 nerves and 650 sweat glands and consists of over 19 million cells.

Skin has two layers:

Epidermis
The outermost layer of skin

Dermis
The layer of skin just below the epidermis. It is the dermis which is richly supplied with blood and nourishes the skin.

Basically the skin is nourished by the lymph fluids that circulate in the internal cellular structure of the skin. This lymph fluid is in constant motion.

**What Is
Healthy Skin**

Healthy skin is one that is elastic and supple. This enables the life-energizing lymph fluid to efficiently fulfill its function . . . nourishing the underlying cellular structure, disposing of the waste products and keeping an alkaline balance.

As one ages, the outer skin layers begin to

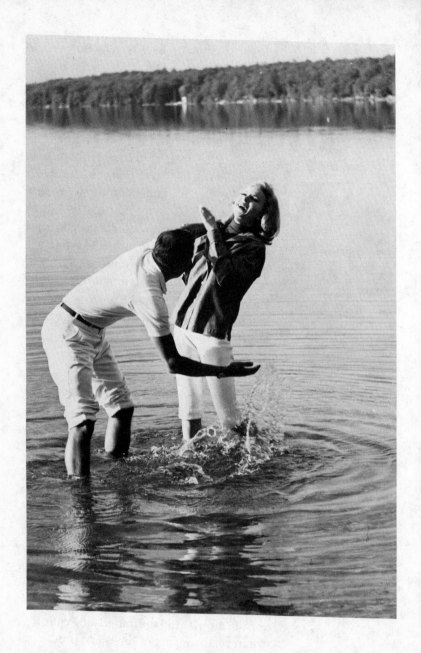

Enjoy the fresh, sparkling skin of your youthful years . . . all through life! Let live juices help give you back that schoolgirl complexion.

thin out . . . veins and tendons on the back of the hand become more pronounced. The skin begins to lose its elasticity. The skin on the forehead, on the cheeks, around the eyes and the chin may start to hang in folds. There is a loss of subcutaneous fat and the skin may appear tight. Aging spots (large brown areas), caused by small hemorrhages which occur under the skin, may become evident.

How To Have Healthy Skin

How can you take care of your skin to assure elasticity and suppleness while keeping it blemish-free? Here are some guidelines:

1. JUICES REJUVENATE SKIN

Dermatitis, dry skin and many other skin blemishes may indicate a vitamin and mineral deficiency.

Carrot juice has been termed an excellent skin food. When juiced and consumed fresh, it is very rich in vital organic alkaline elements such as sodium and potassium. It also contains a good supply of calcium, magnesium and iron.

Cucumber and carrot juice have been found beneficial to skin eruptions; as has raw potato juice.

Green pepper juice (3 ounces) combined with carrot juice (9 ounces) has been found helpful not only to correct skin blemishes but also as an aid to restoring healthy nails and hair.

2. USE COSMETICS SPARINGLY

As I said in the first chapter of this book . . . one or two tablespoons of safflower oil taken inside will do better than applying moisturizers to your face . . . on the outside!

Dry Skin
A Sign Of
Aging

Wrinkles do not come primarily from dry skin. And applying moisturizers is a waste of time. Dry skin is an indication of the aging process . . . but wrinkling is cased by damage to the skin's underlying structure. All a moisturizing cream does is help hold water to your dry skin. This is a temporary measure. But sound nutrition is a more permanent and satisfying measure.

3. AVOID EXCESSIVE EXPOSURE TO THE SUN

Sun bathing is the most damaging way to prematurely age the skin. A 10-minute sun bath at 10 in the morning or 3 in the afternoon is sufficient. Brown may be beautiful at 17 or 21 but you will look like a prune at age 45!

Toners, fresheners, astringents, Castile soap, transparent soap, deodorant soap, soap that floats (or sinks), cocoa butter soap, day creams, night creams, all-purpose creams or ice creams . . . none of these are going to work any miracles to give you that schoolgirl or schoolboy complexion.

Warm Baths
And
Live Juices

Warm baths, a good friction rubdown with a brisk brush or turkish towel and a daily intake of live juices will restore and maintain a healthy, glowing skin . . . the skin you love to touch!

Henry Ward Beecher remarked:

> *Beauty may be said to be*
> *God's trademark in creation.*

Have you looked at your skin lately?

9

HOW TO WIN OVER ARTHRITIS

Arthritis
Is The
World's
Crippler

Over 10% of the world's population have arthritis. Over 60 million Americans suffer from this painful ailment! Of this group 4 million Americans are disabled.

Arthritis in its nearly 100 different forms claims over one-quarter million new victims a year in the United States. It strikes women twice as often as men. And even children fall prey to this ailment.

Arthritis refers to an inflammation of a joint. (Rheumatism is a vague word used for unexplained aches and pains in joints and muscles)

Arthritis, generally, is a link in a chain of ill health. Constipation, accumulation of internal wastes, poor liver function, faulty filtering of the kidneys . . . all can contribute to an arthritic condition.

**Arthritis
A Sign
Of Poor Health**

The use of external medications, ointments, or pain killers does not resolve the problem. It makes one rest in false security. And usually one continues bad eating habits ignoring nature's warning signals . . . until one day that individual is severely crippled with this common ailment.

**Osteoarthritis
Most Common**

The most common type of arthritis is Osteoarthritis. As one gets older it is believed the joint fluid may diminish. The joint fluid is not an oil but a solution of mucous which loses water and thickens under pressure. The point that this fluid comes in contact with on the bone is called the articular cartilage. It grows through childhood, after which it is then formed for life. Cartilage, made up of mucin, albumin and sulfuric acid, is the slippery end of the bone. Osteoarthritis is cartilage destruction.

It is important to keep this cartilage slippery and elastic. Many nutritionists believe this can be done by adding proper oils through correct diet and by keeping a close watch on how calcium enters your body.

**You Do Not
Inherit
Arthritis**

Arthritis is not inherited. What you may inherit are the poor eating habits of your parents . . . thus falling susceptible to the same ailments they had.

You must start rebuilding your body nutri-

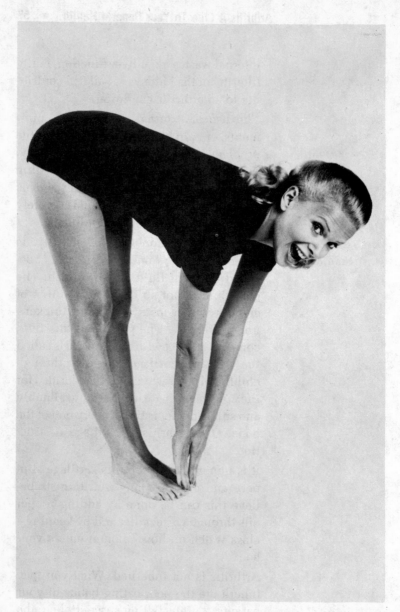

Start an internal cleansing program. At the same time, eliminate bad health habits. Begin live juice therapy. And you may regain the youthful vibrancy and flexibility you once enjoyed in your youth.

tionally from within. I cannot overemphasize this point. Here are some guidelines.

Internal Cleansing

Under your doctor's supervision and approval, fast one day each week. Many people believe a distilled water fast is better than a juice fast for arthritic sufferers; since juices have a high acidity. This is debatable since juices upon consumption, reduce to alkaline nature.

Under supervision have a series of colonics administered to you.

Aid internal cleansing by eating two salads a day . . . not iceberg lettuce, but salads that consist of endive, broccoli, celery, peppers, etc.

Eliminate Bad Habits

Stop smoking, stop drinking both alcoholic beverages and soft drinks. By all means avoid sugar and products that contain sugar such as cakes, pies, and candy. Sugar is particularly injurious to the arthritic, for it causes the walls of the intestines to degenerate and destroys the joint fluid.

Go Easy on Meat

Reduce your meat intake to no more than 3 times a week. And never eat meat that is rare. Broil your meat. Whenever you eat meat, always eat fresh salads with it. Never eat shell fish or fish without scales and stay off of pork products.

Recommended fish are: Mackerel, Sardines, Halibut and Salmon as these con-

How To Get On The Right Road

Three Important Steps To Take

tain the most A and D vitamins.

Never eat fried or scrambled eggs but rather poached or soft boiled eggs. And stay off of coffee and tea. Herb tea is acceptable and beneficial.

Oils to Avoid

Avoid all meat fats and never eat the skin of chicken or any other animal or fowl. Avoid vegetable oils and go easy on nuts. The best oils are found in the fish previously mentioned, in soft boiled or poached eggs, and in natural butter.

Mineral oil, corn oil, cottonseed oil should be avoided.

A Formula That May Help

Dale Alexander is a firm believer in the use of cod liver oil for arthritics. He suggests squeezing the juice from ½ orange (fresh) (or 2 tablespoons of warm, homogenized milk) and one tablespoon of pure cod liver oil. He then suggest you stir for 10-15 seconds and then pour this mixture back and forth between two glasses to create thousands of minute bubbles . . . then drink immediately.

He recommends mixing in two 4-ounce glasses and drinking this just before bedtime and at least 3-4 hours after your evening meal.[1]

Ease off Drugs

Ask your doctor to help you ease off medication as you ease into sound nutrition

[1] Dale Alexander, _Arthritis and Common Sense_, (Connecticut: Witkower Press), 1954, pp. 163-169.

habits. Proper nutrition may help produce natural cortisone in your body as your glands become strengthened.

**Change
Your
Perspective**

Include Juices in Your Diet

Drink 12 ounces at least twice a day of a combination of carrot and celery juice (half and half). Carrots act as a cleanser to cleanse the system of excessive acid and celery contains four times as much organic sodium as it does calcium and is believed highly beneficial for arthritic sufferers.

For a third juice drink during the day, try taking a combination of carrot, apples and beet tops along with a few stalks of celery around 10 AM.

By restoring normal body functions with live foods and juices you may witness arthritic pains and symptoms slowly disappear!

10

HOW TO WIN OVER ULCERS
AND COLITIS

**Fighting
A Disease
That Respects
No Age**

Ulcers and colitis are disease twins and, from a nutritional therapy viewpoint, can be grouped together, as the same treatment applies.

The ulcers discussed in this chapter are the stomach and duodenum ulcers. Ulcers of the stomach are known as <u>gastric</u> ulcers. Ulcers in the duodenum are known as <u>duodenal</u> ulcers.

The duodenum is that segment of the small intestine extending for several inches immediately below the stomach. The duodenal ulcer is the most common form. About one in every ten adults is thought to have a duodenal ulcer! *(One in every 100 adults will have a gastric ulcer.)*

The word *"peptic"* is just a general term used to describe an ulcer.

Most Common Symptoms

The most characteristic symptoms of an ulcer are gnawing hunger pains in the upper abdomen occurring between meals, most often shortly before lunch or supper. What happens is that the lining mucous membrane is eaten away and eroded, leaving a raw, uncovered area in the wall of the stomach or duodenum. Ulcers may vary in size from that of a pinhead to that of a half dollar. Ulcers are not inherited!

A gastric ulcer may turn to cancer. This happens in 1 in 15 cases. Ulcers may rupture and cause severe hemorrhaging.

Ulcers come from bad eating and living habits and a relatively high intake of refined carbohydrates.

A Life Threatening Disease

Colitis, chronic ulcerative colitis, is a life-threatening disease. It is a serious inflammation of the large intestine and is found most often in men and women in the age span of the 30's and 40's.

Those with colitis generally have fever, lose weight, develop anemia and have frequent, bloody, watery bowel movements.[1] The unfortunate victims of chronic ulcera-

---

[1] There may be as many as 20 to 30 movements a day. If this continues one can become dehydrated and develop a high fever.

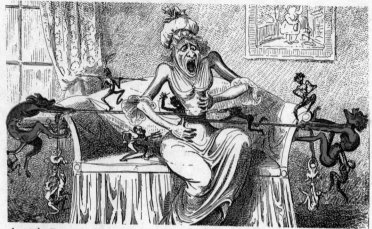

A 19th Century artist portrays a woman seized with internal pains. Those suffering from ulcers or colitis often feel that a war is raging in their abdomen.

tive colitis seem to be highly neurotic and sensitive people. None of the sulfa or antibiotic drugs has been successful in curing this condition.

The Surgical Approach

If the problem persists surgical treatment involves taking a loop of the small intestine out into the abdominal wall and opening it. Intestinal contents then drain out before reaching the diseased large bowel (*colon*). This is called **ileostomy**. If the problem still persists the large bowel is also removed (*colectomy*).

Nutritionists believe it is wise to eliminate solid foods for several days and to go on a liquid diet to regain strength. Then a supervised fast with cleansing enemas are suggested to start the internal housecleaning that is essential for proper healing.

Along with this should be warm or hot baths and an abundance of rest and sleep. Since nervous tension is a contributory factor to both ulcers and colitis, a slower pace of life is of the utmost importance for nature to begin its healing process.

Guidelines For Alleviating The Problem

Raw vegetable juices are a goldmine to anyone who is suffering from ulcers and colitis. Citrus juices should be avoided. When the colon is acutely inflammed, even small portions of food may cause irritation. That is why solid food is not recommended for several days.

Raw vegetable juices become the essential nutrients during this period.

It may seem odd to suggest warm enemas to one suffering from colitis since they may have 20 to 30 movements daily. However, one must remember that the tissues are highly irritated and the warm enemas help remove the putrefying material clinging to the walls of the colon and compounding the problem. It is important, however, that only 2 or 3 glasses of water be used in the cleansing enema!

While milk has been taken for those suffering from stomach ulcers, milk is NOT recommended for colitis.

As one gains strength, finely grated raw vegetables can be added to one's diet.

Cabbage Juice An Effective Agent

In one study, Dr. Garnet Cheney of Stanford University Medical School, San Francisco . . . obtained good results using cabbage juice for ulcers.

Dr. Cheney gave each of 13 patients one quart of cabbage juice, squeezed from fresh, raw cabbages. Those patients who could not tolerate this much cabbage juice were given a combination of 75% cabbage juice with 25% celery juice.

The juice was chilled and five times a day they drank this juice until the quart was exhausted. They were allowed to season it with a little tomato juice.

Foods To Avoid

All fats, pork, fried foods, ice cream were excluded from their diet. They did eat eggs (poached), vegetables and bread made from whole grains.

In the 13 patients, the ulcers disappeared in 12 cases in from six to nine days. One case required 23 days to heal.[1]

What Ulcer Sufferers Need

Ulcer sufferers are deficient in Vitamins C, E and U. Cabbage juice is very high in Vitamin C and also in Vitamin U. Vitamin C helps the blood coagulate, maintains the health of blood vessels and aids the adrenal glands. The adrenal glands are the glands in the body that react to stress. Vitamin E is present in Wheat Germ oil and can also be purchased in capsule form at your health food store.

Raw potato juice is very soothing on the gastric tract and carrot juice is very beneficial.

Juices For Colitis

Many with colitis find relief using the following juice combinations:

Carrot 8 ounces, apple 8 ounces
Carrot 6 ounces, beet 5 ounces
and cucumber 5 ounces

Both ulcers and colitis require a change to a healthy, nutritious diet, an initial juice diet and an elimination of aggravating foods.

---

[1] Dr. L. Newman, *Make Your Juicer Your Drug Store*, (New York: Benedict Lust Publ.), 1970, pp. 70-71.

11

HOW TO WIN
THE BATTLE OF THE BULGE

**Fad
Diets
Will Not
Work!**

The most discouraging thing about middle age is all those years going to waist.

Overweight is sometimes caused by glands, but more often by muscles that enable you to reach for second helpings.

Statistics on the number of people who are overweight are bound to be in round figures.

Worry makes people thin, except when they worry about being fat. Most of us are either too thin to enjoy eating, or too fat to enjoy walking.

How can you win the battle of the bulge? Certainly not by fad diets. They are only temporary measures . . . costly and ineffective.

It has been estimated that 35% of Americans are overweight and the percentage is increasing rapidly.

The Complications of Obesity

Obesity (overweight) is the most common nutritional disorder today in the United States. And the problem with obesity is that it is linked to:

> high blood pressure
> atherosclerosis (clogging arteries)
> diabetes
> strokes

and a host of other ailments. Recognizing these dangers, one who is overweight should be diligent in correcting the problem.

Basic Guidelines To Lose Weight

Most of the popular diets are so drastic that people can't stay on them . . . and they are not very safe nutritionally. Even if you stay on a diet for a month or two, when you come off, you haven't developed any alternate ways of eating. And so you go on a yo-yo sequence.

We are actually eating ourselves to death. We eat far too many calories, yet perform far less physical labor than is necessary to burn up these calories. Just a small difference of 100 calories a day can make a difference of a minimum loss of 10 pounds a year!

Don't pride yourself in eating one meal a

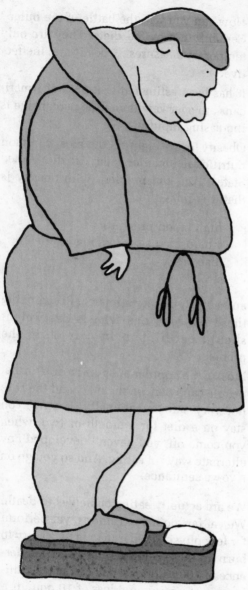

"i wonder
if it was the
maraschino
cherry?"

(Illustration courtesy LIFE & HEALTH)

day. Here are some basic guidelines to follow to successfully fight the battle of the bulge for the rest of your life.

1. Juice Fasting

Read the chapter on juice fasting in this book, and with your doctor's approval, go on a supervised juice fast to bring your weight to an acceptable level.

2. Eat small meals

Once you have done this, do not limit yourself to one large meal daily. Instead try to eat 4 or 5 <u>small</u> meals during the day. And make sure these meals are high in protein and low in carbohydrates and fats.

Housewives and sedentary workers (those who sit at their jobs) use up about 2400 calories a day. To lose weight, the general rule of thumb is to reduce the overall calorie intake to 1200 calories daily. In this way most would lose 1½ pounds a week.

Change
Your
Eating
Habits

3. Avoid hollow calories

Discontinue white bread, white cereals, sugar in any form including cakes, cookies, and candy. Avoid creams and sauces and table salt. Never, never eat those hollow snack foods, such as chips, pretzels, and crackers.

4. Include a daily Juice Diet

You can reduce with juice! And it is essential that you drink live juices daily to insure you're getting the proper nutrients into your system.

When you change your diet from one that is high in carbohydrates and fats, you may go through withdrawal pains. The daily intake of juice will ease you over this healing crisis and carry you steadily to a more svelte you the rest of your life.

While eliminating large calorie intake is important, the source of the calories you eliminate is the most important factor. That is why it is vital to banish from your meals any substantial carbohydrate food. Supplementing the low carbohydrate diet with polyunsaturated fat (*vegetable oil*) increases the oxidation of stored fat (palmitate) by 20 to 25% and aids in diminishing excess weight.

A juice diet is an excellent way to make sure you get the right nutrients while minimizing carbohydrate intake.

Juices That Are Beneficial

Good juice combinations include:

Carrot 8 ounces, celery 8 ounces
Carrot 12 ounces, spinach 4 ounces
Carrot 6 ounces, beet 5 ounces
and cucumber 5 ounces

Vary the juice combinations and drink these 16 ounce drinks 3 or 4 times a day. They will not only supply you with a host of minerals and vitamins but will help eliminate hunger pains and a desire for eating . . . particularly the wrong foods.

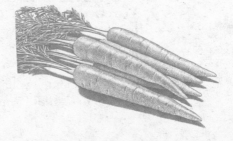

After a supervised fast of four or five days, many have found the following diet beneficial:

Breakfast

A glass of vegetable juice

Fruit Salad

Luncheon

Another large glass of vegetable juice

A large green salad

One boiled or poached egg

Dinner

Steamed, non-starchy vegetables

Broiled liver or other lean meat

Fruit salad

When hungry during the day, try nibbling on strips of raw carrots, celery or pieces of raw cabbage. These are slimming foods as the digestion of raw vegetables burns up more energy than is obtained from them.

12

HOW TO WIN OVER
HIGH BLOOD PRESSURE AND HEART DISEASE

**High
Blood Pressure
A Symptom
Of A Disease**

As we mentioned in an earlier chapter, your body is a vast network of roads. And the interstate highways are the <u>arteries</u> and <u>veins</u>. Arteries all carry blood <u>away</u> from the heart, and veins all carry blood <u>toward</u> the heart.

High blood pressure in itself is not a disease. It is an indication that a disease is present. The medical term for high blood pressure is **HYPERTENSION.**

<u>Hyper</u> means <u>above</u>. Thus the word really means that this is a condition in which the individual has a higher blood pressure than that judged to be normal.

Blood pressure is the result of the force with which the heart pumps the blood

**Understanding
The
Blood Pressure
Scale**

through the arteries of the body. Blood pressure is recorded with two figures:

Systolic pressure - the top figure

Diastolic pressure - the lower figure

<u>Systolic</u> blood pressure is that which is measured when the heart muscle is <u>con</u>-tracting. **Diastolic** blood pressure is that which is measured when the heart muscle <u>relaxes.</u>

In general if the systolic pressure is above 140 or the diastolic above 90, the person is considered to have elevated blood pressure.

It is **NOT** a fact that one's normal blood pressure should be 100 plus the individual's age.

One's blood pressure does tend to rise as one grows older.

**Not In
Favor of
Medication**

Robert E. Rothenberg, M.D. does not believe that people in their sixties, seventies or eighties should always receive medication to lower high blood pressure. He comments:

> This is often not good treatment, as it may lessen the amount of the blood that is pumped to various vital organs. It must not be forgotten that elevated blood pressure often represents a compensatory effort to the heart to pump adequate quantities of oxygen and nutriments through narrowed, sclerotic arteries.[1]

High blood pressure is an indication of possible impending heart disease. The

---

[1] Robert E. Rothenberg, <u>Health in the Later Years,</u> (New York: New American Library), 1964, p. 112.

A blood clot the size of this dot can cause a Heart Attack.

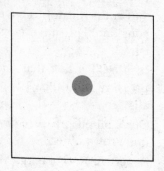

Or a stroke.

Every year, thousands die because of a blood clot. Thousands more become disabled, some permanently.

most common forms of heart disease occur because of one of three conditions:

1. Hypertensive

Hypertensive heart disease is an outcome of blood pressure that is high. The heart must work harder to maintain circulation. To do this the muscle of the heart enlarges. A muscle that enlarges because of too much work placed upon it is eventually sapped of strength and ultimately becomes worn out and damaged. Picture a pipe which becomes encrusted and the tube becomes narrower and narrower. This is called arteriosclerosis *(hardening of the arteries)*. It is this hardening and narrowing of the vessel *"thruway"* that causes the blood pressure to elevate to maintain a sufficient flow of blood for the body. Arteries run the entire length of the body including even to the male and female reproductive organs . . . carrying blood from the heart throughout the body.

2. Coronary Heart Disease

While Hypertensive heart disease is an outcome of blood pressure that is high throughout the circulatory system, coronary heart disease is caused specifically because of a hardening of the coronary (heart) arteries. These are the arteries that supply the heart with blood. This develops slowly and soon the heart is unable to receive an adequate supply of oxygen, and other nutrients.

3. Valvular Heart Disease

Sometimes termed "*rheumatic heart disease*," this heart ailment takes a large toll of human life. The valves of the heart become thickened and scarred. This makes it impossible for them to close or open completely. Normal circulation is disrupted as blood leaks through or is pushed backward.

Diet Important To Recovery

How well each of these diseases will respond to nutritional therapy will depend on how far advanced the disease has progressed.

Here are some basic guidelines many have found beneficial. To a trained medical doctor they may seem simplistic, but nature uses simple approaches to what appear to be complex problems.

Nutritional Supplements

Studies have shown that the lack of Vitamin B6 is one of the causes of weakening of the walls of the arteries. The B-complex vitamins and foods rich in B-complex vitamins may prove beneficial.

The Value Of Vitamin E

Vitamin E both oxygenates the tissues and also has anti-bloodclotting ability. This is important for the heart and the entire arterial system of the body. Vitamin E is also a vasodilator; that is, it opens arteries so that more blood can flow through. This is important to those with hardening of the arteries.

Lecithin is very important for the heart. Many believe that lecithin is a powerful

<u>emulsifying</u> agent. I take two tablespoons at each meal in granular form.

High blood pressure is reported by some to usually respond to a combination of carrot, celery and beet juice . . . with a major portion of the 16 ounce drink made up of celery juice. Some nutritionists recommend drinking two quarts of this combination daily. At the same time as the liquid is taken, garlic capsules are also taken.

Other combinations include drinks of:

Carrot 10 ounces, spinach 6 ounces
Carrot 10 ounces, beet 3 ounces,
cucumber 3 ounces
Carrot 7 ounces, celery 4 ounces,
parsley 2 ounces, spinach 3 ounces

Many times people with high blood pressure eat a lot of salt and salty foods. Doctors urge patients to discontinue these. Also the drugs prescribed often deplete the potassium in one's body. Fruit juices are good sources of replenishing potassium . . . naturally.

13

HOW TO WIN OVER A PESKY PROSTATE

**A Problem
That
Begins In
Middle Age**

The prostate gland is found only in males. It is a solid, flesh-colored, glandular organ, shaped like a horse chestnut. It measures about 1½″ in its three dimensions.

The prostate gland surrounds the neck of the urinary bladder and the beginning of the urethra. The urethra is the channel through which urine passes.

The prostate secretes fluid that comprises a large part of semen. Semen includes sperm cells.

All men over 50 should have their prostates examined every year. When men reach this age, problems of the prostate increase and these problems can be extremely annoying and difficult.

**The Cure
Can Be
Worse
Than The
Problem**

The prostate is often the seat of disorders which often end in surgical correction. Sometimes the "cure" is worse than the problem.

Among the prostate problems that can occur are the following:

1. Infection

This is called prostatitis. The symptoms include high temperature, back pain, frequent and painful urination.

2. Prostate enlargment (Benign)

As men approach 40 the prostate generally undergoes enlargment. When the prostate enlarges it presses on the neck of the urinary bladder and obstructs the outflow of urine. As the problem progresses, there is a decrease in the size and force of the urinary stream. Residual urine remains in the bladder. Kidney function decreases and, if not corrected, kidney failure and uremia (*a toxic condition*) will ensue. Other complications can be bladder stone formation and infection. If at any point you find yourself unable to void or can only pass just a few drops of urine . . . you should contact your doctor immediately. Such a condition demands surgical action.

Don't
Be A
Statistic

3. Cancer of the prostate

Cancer of the prostate generally occurs in those beyond 60 years of age. Cancer of the prostate is the most common malignancy in the male. It is estimated that approximately one out of four men will develop cancer of the prostate before they reach 70. There are no early warning signs.

4. Stones in the Prostate Gland (calculi)

Stones can be diagnosed by your doctor in his normal examination of the prostate. Prostate stones can cause an obstruction in the flow of urine.

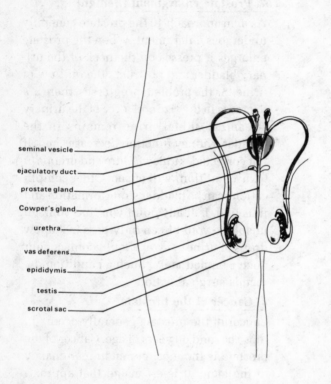

seminal vesicle

ejaculatory duct

prostate gland

Cowper's gland

urethra

vas deferens

epididymis

testis

scrotal sac

Prostate problems generally evidence themselves with a constant feeling of fullness in the bladder and with frequent, urgent trips to the bathroom. One cannot sleep through the night without getting up and going to the bathroom.

Almost 80% of men over 60 years of age suffer from an enlarged prostate. Enlargment of the prostate does not interfere with sexual relations; however, such relations may diminish when one experiences the uncomfortable symptoms it displays.

The Medical Approach

Medically, prostate problems are treated with antibiotics and relaxant drugs. When this fails, surgery is employed.

There are several types of surgery used. When possible, it is best to avoid surgery and not allow your condition to progress to this stage. Some surgical methods are:

1. Suprapubic prostatectomy

The bladder is opened and drained and the prostate gland removed.

2. Retropubic prostatectomy

The prostate gland is removed directly, without opening the bladder, by making an incision in the lower part of the abdomen. Sometimes the incision is made in front of the rectum (perineal prostatectomy).

3. Transurethral prostatectomy

No incision is made. The obstructing portion of the prostate is cut away by an electrically charged wire loop which is inserted through the penis.

Several modes of nutritional therapy have

been tried with gratifying success. They include:

1. Vitamin F (unsaturated fatty acids)

This has been beneficial in helping to completely empty the bladder. Many have noticed decrease in fatigue and increase in sexual urge.

2. Vitamins A and E and Amino acids

Many acknowledge the restorative powers of Vitamin A and the ability of Vitamin E to help the reproductive tract.

The three amino acids recommended — alanine, glutamic acid and glycine are rich in protein and are best found in soybeans and peanuts.

3. Pumpkin seeds

Dr. W. Devrient, a German doctor, remarks:

> *Only the plain people knew the open secret of pumpkin seeds; they all knew that pumpkin seeds preserve the prostate gland and thereby, male potency.*

I personally take one pumpkin seed oil capsule daily at breakfast.

4. Zinc

The prostate gland, when normal, contains more zinc than any other organ in the body. An ailing prostate has a deficient supply of zinc. Whole eggs, onions, oatmeal, peas, beans, and beef liver are particularly high in zinc.

Cucumber, carrot and beet juice represent one of the finest cleansing and healing juice combinations for the prostate and sex glands.

The Nutritional Approach

The Value Of Pumpkin Seeds

Zinc And Juices

14

HOW TO IMPROVE YOUR EYESIGHT

**Eyesight
Problems
Begin At An
Early Age**

Benjamin Franklin once said:

Keep your eyes wide open before marriage, and half-shut afterwards.

While Victor Hugo remarked:

Men have sight; women insight.

Some teenagers claim to have excellent vision . . . love at first sight. The cure for love at first sight . . . is second sight.

Seriously though, more and more youngsters are having eye problems and poor nutrition is a contributing factor.

**Eyes
Abound
In Nerve Cells**

More nerve cells are devoted to serving our sense of sight than are devoted to any of our other senses. Therefore, it is important that these nerve cells are constantly bathed in proper nourishment.

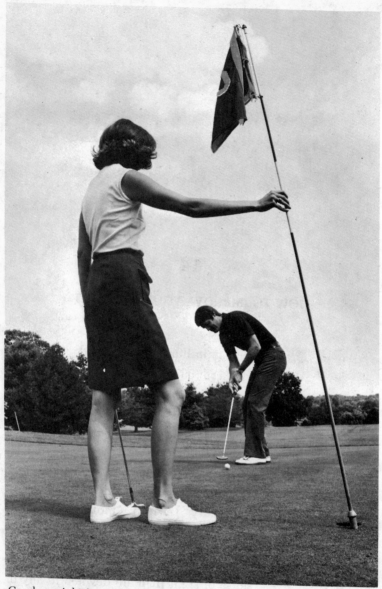

Good eyesight is a precious possession. It enables you to fully enjoy the pleasures of life, whether on the golf course, or sharing in a family reunion. Sound nutrition practices will help you retain and improve this precious possession.

At the rear of each eye is a thick optic nerve which passes to the visual cortex of the brain. The eye rotates using six external ocular muscles.

The eyeball has three major coats:

1. The smooth, protective outer sclera
2. The middle, pigmented choroid
3. The inner, light-sensitive retina

The sclera is the "*white*" of the eye. In the cornea of the eye lies the lens. In front of the lens is a circular muscular diaphragm, the iris, which gives the eye its color. Our vision is accomplished in a way similar to taking a picture with a camera.

Light rays from the object pass through the cornea, the pupil, the lens and finally reach the retina. When light hits the light-sensitive cells of the retina, they stimulate the nerve cells. The optic nerve carries the message to the seeing part of the brain (*visual cortex*).

Some eye defects include:

Eye Problems Are Many

1. Nearsightedness (Myopia)

The light rays are focused before they reach the retina; thus a person can see objects near him well while not being able to focus on objects that are at a far distance.

2. Astigmatism

Astigmatism occurs when one of the components of the lens system becomes egg-shaped rather than spherical. Therefore a person is unable to focus any object clearly, regardless how far or near it is. Sight becomes blurred.

3. Farsightedness (Hypermetropia)

Caused by failure of the lens to bend the light rays enough to bring them to a focal point on the retina. One can see distant objects better than objects that are close.

Diseases of the eye include:

Glaucoma

This results from an increase of pressure inside the eyeball. This pressure slowly destroys the optic nerve unless corrective measures are taken. Otherwise, blindness will be the final outcome.

Cataract

The lens, which is normally transparent, may become milky and opaque in older persons. This limits adequate light reaching the retina. Vision becomes blurred. An operation removes this clouded lens.

Retinitis Pigmentosa

This is characterized by a slow but eventual total degeneration of the retina and causes blindness in thousands of Americans annually. It is preceded by years of night blindness.

Nutrition's
Answer
To
Eye Problems

Generally, many of the eye problems are caused by some form of nutritional deficiency. Carrots have always been known as the "eye" vegetable; the reason being that they are so rich in Vitamin A. And Vitamin A is essential for the eyes.

One comedian said that he took so much carrot juice that when he went to bed at night he could see through his closed eyelids!

It must be remembered that the eyes are merely the indication of the health level of the entire body. Trouble in any part of the body can show up in defective eyesight.

Anyone seeking to correct defective vision should go on a program of good cleansing and rebuilding . . . nutritionally.

A good cleansing begins with a supervised fast and a change to a sound nutritional diet. Commercial teas, coffee, cocoa or alcoholic beverages should be avoided.

Raw Salads And Vitamin E

Raw salads should be eaten daily . . . particularly those raw vegetables rich in Vitamin A. Weaknesses in eye muscles, crossed eyes, blurred vision, have been alleviated by taking Vitamin E or liver and yeast. Night blindness is due to a Vitamin A deficiency. And carrot juice can be helpful. Vitamin A deficiency can also cause extreme muscular weakness.

Carrot Juice Daily

Nutritionists recommend Carrot juice daily; about 2 quarts, as a lack of Vitamin A is responsible for many eye ailments. Some combinations include:

Carrot 12 ounces, spinach 4 ounces
Carrot 8 ounces, celery 8 ounces
Carrot 8 ounces, celery 6 ounces
Spinach 2 ounces

Fennel juice has also been found to be beneficial. Fennel is a member of the parsley family and resembles celery.

Parsley juice is also used. It must be remembered that parsley juice is very potent. Therefore only one tablespoon of juice should be taken at a time. It is best mixed in with carrot juice.

Eliminate Stress

Glaucoma is often induced by stress and daily juice intake of carrot and celery juice helps relieve stressful attitudes while building up the eye (and the rest of the body) nutritionally.

Better eyesight begins with better nutrition!

15

HOW TO WIN OVER CONSTIPATION

Clogged Colons And Sticky Buns

It has often been said that America is the land of clogged colons!

Is it any wonder? Recall the food you ate over the past 24 hours. Did it include a greasy hamburger nestled in a soft bun, french fries, coffee and pie?

How much of the food you ate was as Nature prepared it . . . _raw_? **The most perfect food is food as it grows.**

When food manufacturers get hold of it, they cook it to death, add back color artificially, and then can it. If one wants food as close to its peak (outside of fresh picking) frozen food is the best buy nutritionally.

The Headache Twins . . . Constipation and Diarrhea

With the highly processed foods we buy and very little roughage that we eat, millions of people suffer from irregular bowel habits and constipation or diarrhea.

Many doctors believe that over 75% of ailments have their start in an unhealthy colon.

**Trouble
On the
Thruway**

Picture your body as a thruway. You eat food. It is transported through your stomach, then to the small intestines and large intestines (colon) and finally the residue is eliminated. While this illustration is over-simplified, imagine what happens when, after years of misuse, the muscles of the colon become tired, flabby and sluggish. Add to this deadly wastes clinging to the walls of the colon and accumulating for years into disease-breeding pockets. As the colon becomes clogged, everything backs up.

That which cannot be eliminated then starts to slowly seep back up the system to the intestines, the stomach, the lungs, the breasts. And soon you notice a multitude of vague ailments that you just can't put your finger on . . . hints that your body is rebelling from years of misuse.

Like a thruway, when an accident occurs, traffic backs up for miles . . . and does not get moving again until the cause of the accident is removed.

**Harsh
Laxatives
Are Dangerous**

With a clogged-up kitchen sink, you can pour "*Drano*" in it and clear it up in a hurry. Your body is far more delicate. And the taking of harsh laxatives over the years acts like a whip. They do not allow the colon to perform its normal peristaltic (*wave-like*) propelling function. Soon you have a tiger by the tail.

Constipation gives birth or contributes to a host of diseases including: diabetes, obesity, epilepsy, gall bladder problems, ulcers, arthritis and vascular problems such as high blood pressure and heart trouble. **A large majority of ill people have one thing in common . . . *poor bowel habits.*** And the very first step towards recovery should include a change in diet to fresh, raw foods and juices (at least 2 pints daily) to get the colon unclogged and the poisons flowing out and to revitalize a devitalized, undernourished body.

Your body should become a gentle, flowing stream but if your body more resembles a stagnant pool, you are courting illness.

If you are eating all the wrong foods and have bowel movements daily, <u>don't</u> assume your bowels are functioning normally. This is not necessarily the case. Many persons have daily bowel movements, yet they suffer from constipation and sluggishness. The muscles of the colon may propel the waste material slowly and some may settle into pockets or cling to the colon walls because of a highly refined diet. Waste, coming through, passes by this slimy or encrusted wall, not picking up the aged waste. Thus, you have a movement and falsely believe, your bowels are healthy.

Many doctors disagree as to how long residue can remain in the bowel. Some do not get alarmed if an individual only has a movement once or twice a week. Nutritionists would disagree with this thinking. Many believe that if poisonous residue remains as long as 48 to 72 hours it can

Is Your Body a Stagnant Pool?

Daily Bowel Movements May Not Be A Sign of Good Health

How Often Should You Have a Bowel Movement?

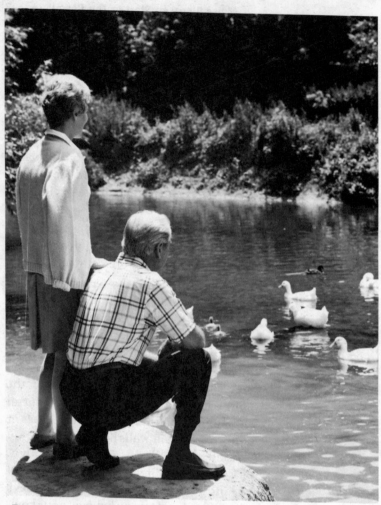

Determine right now to wake up that sluggish colon. Turn it from a stagnant pool into a gentle, flowing stream.

be a source of internal problems. A bowel movement twice a day is considered by many to be ideal.

One should find that in like proportion as you eliminate highly processed junk foods from your diet and switch over to live foods and juices, the bowels will regulate themselves to what is normal for you. **The number of movements is not as important as the diet.** It's the correct diet that makes the difference.

Many have found that immediately upon arising (before brushing your teeth) that the drinking of liquids is beneficial for normal movements. Six to 8 ounces of water with the juice of one-half lemon and/or two tablespoons of granular lecithin is highly productive and also very stimulating.

Hints For A Flowing Stream

In my daily morning juice drink (described in a previous chapter), I include the juice of one pear. The pear is a natural laxative, and has a host of minerals that many believe nourishes the male prostate gland and is insurance against future problems.

Pectin In Apples Beneficial

I also include in my daily juice drink, an apple. Apples contain **pectin.** Pectin is a detoxifying agent and promotes the normal passage of food wastes through the colon, without harsh, irritating effects while also becoming an aid in reducing blood cholesterol levels. (*One to four tablespoons of scraped apple, given every hour, is sometimes used for diarrhea.*)

Enemas and Colonics

Colonics and enemas are emergency means to correct diseased colons so a live food diet can be of value. They should not be relied on permanently but only to get the thruway back into operation. Most doctors do not favor either colonics or enemas but lean towards drugs and possibly surgery. Nutritionists believe, for the most part, in the use of colonics and enemas.

A colonic irrigation involves injecting into the colon a large amount of water, flowing in and flushing out to wash out material situated above the defecation area and to wash the wall of the bowel as high as the water can be made to reach. Generally a series of 6-12 colonics are given to remove the encrustations of the colon and empty out the pockets. A colonic is not painful and the end result may be both rewarding and refreshing.

Juice combinations many have found beneficial for constipation include:

Carrot 8 ounces, apple 8 ounces

Carrot 8 ounces, celery 4 ounces, apple 4 ounces

How is your colon? Is it part of a gentle, flowing stream or is it a stagnant pool? Live foods and live juices **can** make a vibrant difference!

16

HOW TO KEEP SLIM AND YOUNG
WITH JUICE FASTING

**Fasting,
The
Royal Road
To Healing**

In my book, How To Keep Healthy &
Happy by Fasting[1], I discuss in detail both
the history and benefits as well as the
methods of fasting.

This chapter will only touch on the high-
lights of juice fasting, in particular.

Fasting should be done under proper medical supervision. Dr. Otto H. F. Buchinger,
Jr., a medical doctor, believes that fasting
is *the Royal Road to Healing.* I would
agree with him.

Particularly in America we subsist, for the
most part, on a nutritional Titanic that

---

[1] Salem Kirban, How To Keep Healthy & Happy by
Fasting, (Salem Kirban, Inc., Kent Road, Huntingdon Valley, Pennsylvania 19006) $2.95 plus 50¢
for postage.

**Our
Nutritional
Titanic**

gives host to myriad ailments. Proper fasting becomes a broom that sweeps clean our digestive and eliminative processes and by so doing prevents or eliminates diseases.

Fasting does not cure anything. It is a cleansing process which enables the body to heal itself. There are at least 15 specific instances in the Bible where people fasted.

**Fasting
A
Cleansing
Process**

At age 50 I underwent a 3-day supervised fast with heartwarming results. I personally found it very beneficial. And I have been enjoying the fruits of this fast since.

However, I must caution you, that to fast and then go back to your old eating habits will prove disappointing. After I fasted for three days, I then changed my eating habits relying as much as possible on live foods and live juices and eliminating highly processed foods, sweets and desserts. A fast can steer you on the road to good health. **But to stay on that road, one must fuel the body with live foods.**

Many believe that fasting is one of the safest healing methods known.

**My
3-Day
Fast
Successful**

My 3-day fast consisted of drinking 4 ounces of distilled water on the half-hour and 4 ounces of lemon water on the hour. I did this daily for 3 days from 9 AM until 8 PM. (Again, may I caution you not to attempt a fast without proper medical supervision, preferably at a reputable, recognized retreat)

Some nutritionists believe **juice** fasting is a more effective cleansing agent. Juice fast-

Juice
Fasting vs.
Water
Fasting

ing also results in much faster recovery and rejuvenation of the tissues.

They recommend juice fasting because raw juices are rich in minerals, vitamins, enzymes and trace elements; and they are very easily assimilated. They believe these juices are vital to normalizing all the body processes and aid in speedy cell regeneration.

At some juice fasting clinics, enemas are given daily and colonics once a week to loosen and discharge the pockets of old, hardened fecal matter that is almost cemented to the walls of the colon.

How To
Break
A Fast

Breaking the fast properly is just as important as the fast. You ease off a fast slowly. If you have fasted for 3 days, the following 3 days should be a gradual restoration of eating. One should eat very slowly.

First day after a 3-day Fast

> Broth for breakfast
> > (made up of carrots, potato skins, beets and celery tops)
> Salad and juice for lunch
> Salad, juice and broth for supper

On the second day, you can **add** soaked prunes or figs for breakfast, drinking the soaking liquid as well; and perhaps two small apples between meals plus the same menu as recommended for Day One.

For the third day, one can eat all the items previously mentioned and **add** a container of plain yogurt for breakfast, **add** a baked potato for lunch and **add** a whole-grain

Types of Juice Fasts

bread with cheese for supper.

Many nutritionists have recommended certain juices to use in a juice fast for specific conditions. Some believe these juices should be taken every half-hour from upon arising to retiring in 4-ounce units.

For purifying and cleansing one's body

Fruit juices, (freshly juiced) and juice of carrot, celery, beets, cabbage, beet tops, a few sprigs of parsley

For arthritis

Vegetable juices such as: carrot, celery and alfalfa, beets and beet tops. Some drink over 1 pint of celery juice daily.

For prostate problems

Vegetable and fruit juices such as: apples, pears, kale, carrots, asparagus and cucumber.

For overweight

Vegetable and fruit juices such as: watercress, celery, parsley, lemon, pineapple and grape.

For nervousness and insomnia

Fresh juices such as: carrots, celery and lettuce.

For emphysema

Raw juices such as: watercress, carrots, parsnips, potatoes, lemons and black currants.

For asthma

Raw juices such as: comfrey, horse radish, garlic, carrot, celery and lemon.

**High Blood
Pressure
And a
Fast**

Paavo O. Airola, a nutritionist and naturopath states:

> The best thing to do for high blood pressure is to go on a juice fast ... The most suitable juices for high blood pressure are citrus fruits, black currants and grapes, plus carrots, spinach, comfrey, parsley, onions and garlic (as an addition) ... For **edema**, or water-logged body tissues, juices of pears and dandelions are used.[1]

A doctor will adapt juice fasting therapy to meet the requirements of each individual case. The juice combinations described have only been given for general information and should in **no way** be construed as prescribing for cases of illness. Show these pages to your doctor and ask him to advise you and supervise your raw juice therapy.

---

[1] Paavo O. Airola, How To Keep Slim, Healthy, and Young with Juice Fasting, (Arizona: Health Plus Publishers), 1971, pp. 57, 58.

17

HOW TO HAVE A SECOND HONEYMOON
EVERY DAY FOR THE REST OF YOUR LIFE

A Brief Period of Apparent Agreement

Marriage was ordained by God and designed to fill basic needs of mankind.

The dictionary defines the word, "Honeymoon" as:

> a brief period of apparent agreement, as between political parties after an election.

God recognized man's need for a partner and said:

> It is not good for the man to be alone; I will make him a helper suitable for him.

> (Genesis 2:18)

To Walk Side by Side

The problems in marriage sometimes arise because man does not accept the fact that woman came from his rib *(to walk by his side)* and **not** his foot *(to be stepped upon).*

It may sometimes get trying for a man when his newly wed wife doesn't turn on the stove. She just lights the grease. Some wives need plastic surgery . . . the removal of all their credit cards.

Sometimes like Jacob, you are in for a surprise. One person remarked:

> The way my wife looks in the morning!
> She ran after the garbage man and said,
>   "Am I too late for the garbage?"
> He said,
>   "No, jump in."

When the Honeymoon Is Over

The honeymoon is the period between "I do" and "You'd better!"

And many a young bride soon learns that marriage begins when you sink in his arms and ends with your arms in the sink!

The average wife remembers when and where she got married. What escapes her is why.

Some couples are celebrating their Tin Anniversary . . . 12 years eating out of cans.

True Love Unquenchable

The greatest Biblical love story is the Song of Solomon. Solomon knew well both the joys of marriage and the sorrows of adultery. In portraying the attractions between man and woman, Solomon wrote:

> Many waters cannot quench love,
> Nor will rivers overflow it;
> If a man were to give all the riches of
>   his house for love,
> It would be utterly despised.
>   (The Song of Solomon 8:7)

Paul recognized the sexual needs within the marital union and outlined both the husband and wife's responsibility in the New Testament book of 1 Corinthians, chapter 7.

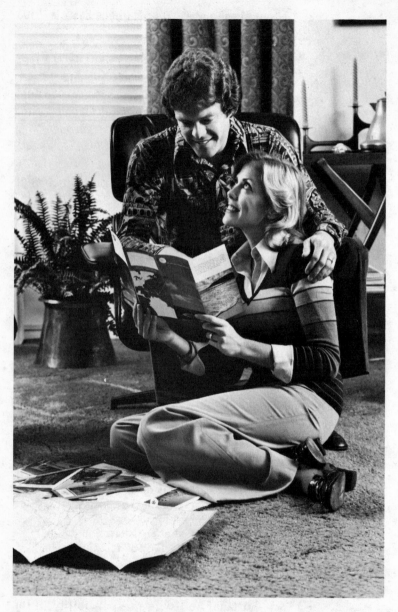

Live juices, taken faithfully each day by both husband and wife, can make a marriage a continuous honeymoon. It will be like a travel adventure where each day brings new joys and happiness!

Someone once remarked that the world's greatest optimists are found at the marriage license bureau. Weddings are certainly a happy occasion. But the joy can be very short-lived.

**From
Mountaintop
to
Valley**

Witness the widespread marital problems that soon surface, the rash of divorces. If one marries for lust instead of love, soon the joy becomes jaded and the mountaintop thrills become valleys of despair.

That honeymoon . . . that brief period of agreement . . . soon ends, and the storms of life ensue.

**Roadblocks
To a
Happy Marriage**

Today's world offers many more roadblocks to a successful and happy marriage than the world of 20 or 30 years ago. Some of the problems a young married couple face include:

1. The increasing difficulty of meeting normal, day to day expenses, in the light of escalating inflation.

2. The new standards of living which tend to make us think of certain material goods as necessities (that were once thought of as luxuries).

3. The new morality and permissiveness that destroys the holy bond of marriage.

4. The increasing deterioration of the foods we eat coupled with the development of poor eating habits with the advent of fast-food fare restaurants.

This chapter primarily deals with point No. 4, our diet. As a husband and wife get older, their honeymoon vigor and vitality can quickly diminish if their nutrition habits are poor.

Fatigue, Fighting and **Fear** are three barriers to a happy marriage.

Fatigue can be generated because of poor eating habits. And in the Hamburger and French Fry America, this is a common disorder. Fatigue then develops into lack of patience, short tempers and constant bickering and **fighting**. And as ailments slowly creep into your life, **Fear** takes over . . . (for the man) fear of losing your manhood, (for the women) fear of losing your beauty.

**Three Steps
To a
Happy Marriage**

From a physical standpoint, here are the steps necessary to have a second honeymoon every day for the rest of your life:

1. **Eliminate Junk Foods**

   Stay off of those hamburgers, french fries, all fried foods, all candy, all sugary desserts, all pork products, all shellfish, all soft drinks.

2. **Eat Live Foods**

   Live foods for live bodies. Eat two fresh salads twice a day. Not iceberg lettuce salads but salads made up of endive, Romaine lettuce, parsley, carrots, celery, radishes, etc. Nibble on carrots or celery sticks between meals rather than candy or cookies.

3. **Drink Live Juices**

   Drink 16 ounces of live juices twice a day (breakfast and about 2:30 PM). If you are a man, include a pear with your morning juice.

Advice
That Works

If you are planning to follow this just for a week or two and expect a miracle . . . forget it! Mother Nature works slowly but effectively. I have followed this advice and I know it works!

To you, it may seem oversimplified. But if you start with sound nutritional practices to rejuvenate a tired, worn-out body, you are starting on the right foot towards having a second honeymoon every day for the rest of your life.

Coupled with this are spiritual guidelines you must follow for true marital happiness. Find your family Bible, dust it off, read it and apply its advice in your life. You can bring back the joy of that honeymoon . . . a honeymoon that will last the rest of your life!

Bibliography

Adams, Ruth and Murray, Frank, *All You Should Know About Beverages*, Larchmont Books, New York, 1976.

Airola, Paavo O., *How To Keep Slim With Juice Fasting*, Health Plus, Publishers, Arizona, 1971.

Charmine, Susan E., *The Complete Raw Juice Therapy*, Baronet Publishing Company, New York, 1977.

Lust, John B., *Raw Juice Therapy*, Thorsons Publishers Limited, England, 1959.

Newman, Dr. L., *Make The Juicer Your Drug Store*, Benedict Lust Publications, New York, 1970.

Null, Gary and Null, Steve, *The Complete Handbook of Nutrition*, Dell Publishing Company, New York 1972.

Walker, N.W., *Raw Vegetable Juices*, Pyramid Books, New York, 1975.

HOW TO EAT YOUR WAY BACK TO

VIBRANT HEALTH

by Salem Kirban

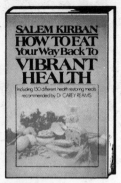

Includes 147 different health restoring
meals that will add variety and vitality
both to you and your family!

FULL COLOR PHOTOS $3.95

Answers These Questions and Many More . . .

- How much water should I drink daily?
- Why is juice so important for sound nutrition?
- Should I drink carrot juice or green drink?
- What foods should I never eat?
- What is the key to selecting the right foods to eat?
- How can I restore my energy and eliminate fatigue?
- Why is Reserve Energy the key to good health or illness?
- When should I take vitamins? Minerals?
- How can I begin a simple, day by day health program?
- What physical changes should I anticipate?
- How much should I eat and when should I eat?
- How can I check my own Nutrition Profile daily?
- Why are celery and lettuce so important?
- Why can't some people assimilate Vitamin C?
- What diet can take you out of the heart attack zone?
- How does urine give you a picture of your current health?
- Why is Lemon Water a miracle drink?
- Ten mistakes people make in eating!
- How your mirror can give you a health profile!
- Coffee or tea . . . which is the greater poison?
- What foods contribute to serious illness?
- Allergies? The *simple* way to determine your allergy!
- What meats may destroy the health of your family?
- How you can conquer constipation . . . diarrhea.
- How can I feel like 20 at 60?
- How can I turn my marriage into a honeymoon?

EXTRA BONUS! THREE-DAY TURN AROUND DIET!
Salem Kirban has included in this book a "How To" section that will
show you, <u>step by step</u>, how to turn around your body chemistry
towards better health . . . in just 3 days. Most people find this <u>TURN
AROUND DIET</u> gives them a new vibrancy and a feeling of well being . . .
fatigue disappears, they lose unwanted weight . . . the sun starts to
shine again! **It's almost like finding the Fountain of Youth!**

Use this ORDER FORM to order additional copies of

HOW JUICES RESTORE HEALTH NATURALLY

by Salem Kirban

You will want to share
these life-sustaining
ideas with your loved
ones and friends.

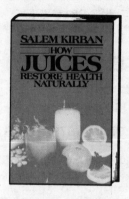

FULL COLOR
Easy-to-read
TYPE!

PRICES

1 copy: $4.95
3 copies: $12 (You save $2.85)
7 copies: $24.50 (You save $10.15)
12 copies: $36.00 (You save $23.40)

WE PAY POSTAGE!

ORDER FORM

SALEM KIRBAN, Inc.
Kent Road
Huntingdon Valley, Penna. 19006 U.S.A.

Enclosed find $ _____ for _____ copies of **HOW JUICES RESTORE HEALTH NATURALLY** by Salem Kirban.

Ship postage paid to:

Name _____
(Please PRINT)

Street _____

City _____

State _____ Zip Code _____

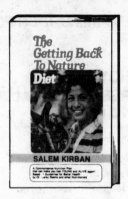
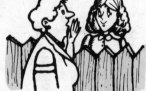

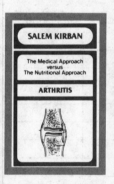 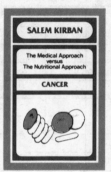 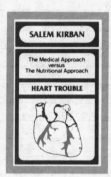 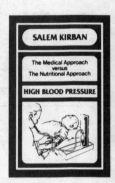

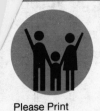

Salem Kirban Family Catalog Order Form

Salem Kirban, Inc.
Kent Road, Huntingdon Valley, Penna. 19006

Please Print

Mr./Mrs./Miss _____

Address _____

City _____ State _____ Zip _____

Name of Item	Qty.	Price Each	Total Price
		Total	
		Add PACKING charge	$1.00
		TOTAL PAYMENT enclosed	

SHARE YOUR HAPPINESS WITH A FRIEND

Do you have friends or relatives who are interested in nutrition and gifts
that uplift and bring joy? Let us send them a 1-year subscription to our
FAMILY CATALOG **free!** Just print their names and addresses below.

Mr.
Miss
Mrs. _____

Mr.
Miss
Mrs. _____

Address _____

Address _____

City _____ State _____ ZIP

City _____ State _____ ZIP

100% GUARANTEE! When you buy from us…you become a part of our
family. We will give you a full refund on every item returned unused!